DISCONNECTED KIDS

DISCONNECTED KIDS

The Groundbreaking Brain Balance Program

for Children with Autism, ADHD, Dyslexia,

and Other Neurological Disorders

Dr. Robert Melillo

A PERIGEE BOOK

A PERIGEE BOOK
Published by the Penguin Group
Penguin Group (USA) Inc.
375 Hudson Street, New York, New York 10014, USA

Penguin Group (Canada), 90 Eglinton Avenue East, Suite 700, Toronto, Ontario M4P 2Y3, Canada
    (a division of Pearson Penguin Canada Inc.)
Penguin Books Ltd., 80 Strand, London WC2R 0RL, England
Penguin Group Ireland, 25 St. Stephen's Green, Dublin 2, Ireland (a division of Penguin Books Ltd.)
Penguin Group (Australia), 250 Camberwell Road, Camberwell, Victoria 3124, Australia
    (a division of Pearson Australia Group Pty. Ltd.)
Penguin Books India Pvt. Ltd., 11 Community Centre, Panchsheel Park, New Delhi—110 017, India
Penguin Group (NZ), 67 Apollo Drive, Rosedale, North Shore 0632, New Zealand
    (a division of Pearson New Zealand Ltd.)
Penguin Books (South Africa) (Pty.) Ltd., 24 Sturdee Avenue, Rosebank, Johannesburg 2196,
    South Africa
Penguin Books Ltd., Registered Offices: 80 Strand, London WC2R 0RL, England

While the author has made every effort to provide accurate telephone numbers and Internet addresses at the time of publication, neither the publisher nor the author assumes any responsibility for errors, or for changes that occur after publication. Further, the publisher does not have any control over and does not assume any responsibility for author or third-party websites or their content.

PRINTING HISTORY
Perigee hardcover edition / January 2009
Perigee trade paperback edition / January 2010

Perigee trade paperback ISBN: 978-0-399-53560-4

The Library of Congress has cataloged the Perigee hardcover edition as follows:

Melillo, Robert.
  Disconnected kids : the groundbreaking brain balance program for children with autism, ADHD, dyslexia, and other neurological disorders / Robert Melillo.— 1st ed.
     p. cm.
  Includes index.
  ISBN 978-0-399-53475-1
  1. Pediatric neurology. 2. Brain-damaged children—Treatment.
3. Children—Diseases. 4. Nervous system—Diseases. I. Title.
  RJ486.M44 2009
  618.92'8—dc22   2008036482

PRINTED IN THE UNITED STATES OF AMERICA

10   9   8   7   6   5

PUBLISHER'S NOTE: Neither the publisher nor the author is engaged in rendering professional advice or services to the individual reader. The ideas, procedures, and suggestions contained in this book are not intended as a substitute for consulting with your physician. All matters regarding your health require medical supervision. Neither the author nor the publisher shall be liable or responsible for any loss or damage allegedly arising from any information or suggestion in this book.

Most Perigee books are available at special quantity discounts for bulk purchases for sales promotions, premiums, fund-raising, or educational use. Special books, or book excerpts, can also be created to fit specific needs. For details, write: Special Markets, Penguin Group (USA) Inc., 375 Hudson Street, New York, New York 10014.

CONTENTS

ACKNOWLEDGMENTS

I DEDICATE THIS book first and foremost to my wife, Carolyn, and my children, Robby, Ellie, and Ty—I love you all, you are my life's true inspiration and the foundation of all I am and all I do. Second, to my parents, Catherine and Joseph, for all their love and support. Third, to my sister, Susan, and my brother, Domenic, and all of their families: Bill, Susan, Billy, Jeffrey, Katie, Colleen, Joey, Alexandra, Olivia, and Nick. You all have played a role in this accomplishment, and I love you all. I would like to thank Ted Carrick and Gerry Leisman for their professional inspiration and support, and Debora Yost for all her help, advice, expertise, and patience. Last but not least, I would like to thank my agent, Carol Mann, and her staff, and all those in my Brain Balance family, especially my nephew and partner, Billy Fowler, as well as Chris, Mike, Peter, Gary, and Susanne. You have all helped greatly in the development of this book, the Brain Balance Program, and the Brain Balance Centers. A special thanks to Denise Festa, who started me on this journey all those years ago.

INTRODUCTION

Stopping the Worst Childhood Epidemic of Our Time

■

I keep on picturing all these little kids playing some game in this big field of rye and all. Thousands of little kids, and nobody's around—nobody big, I mean— except me. I'm standing on the edge of some crazy cliff. What I have to do, I have to catch everybody if they start to go over the cliff. I mean if they're running and they don't look where they're going I have to come out from some- where and catch them. That's all I'd do all day. I'd just be the catcher in the rye and all. I know it's crazy, but that's the only thing I'd really like to be."

—J. D. SALINGER, *THE CATCHER IN THE RYE*

■

WE LIVE IN a world and a time of great contradiction. On the one hand, we are experiencing unprecedented advances in technology. The world's information is literally at our fingertips. We can access high-tech entertainment on a giant screen in a flash. We can communicate with anyone anywhere in the world by flipping open a cell phone.

Yet at the same time, we are experiencing an alarming escalation in the number of children who cannot fully function in this world because they don't have fully functioning brains. Today there are some 16 million chil- dren who are diagnosed with severe attention, behavioral, and learning problems. Every day thousands more are being diagnosed with ADHD, autism, Asperger's syndrome, dyslexia, Tourette syndrome, obsessive-compulsive disorder, bipolar disorder, or other frightening conditions that confirm that something is not right in the brain.

This is a new phenomenon and the most important health issue of our time. Just ten years ago, autism was considered a rare disorder that was diagnosed in about 1 out of every 10,000 children born in the United States. Now, 1 out of 150 children will be diagnosed with autism. Other conditions are skyrocketing at a similar rate. These statistics are making headline news everywhere because doctors, scientists, and concerned parents want answers. Why is this happening? How can we stop it? What can we do about it?

I began searching for these answers nearly fifteen years ago when I started hearing about and reading about these statistics. I saw then, as I still do now, that our community of scientists, doctors, therapists, and educators has been missing something. We have been addressing and treating childhood neurological disorders the same way since the 1950s. Obviously, we haven't been doing it right! I speak to parent and teacher groups all the time and have found that most parents, teachers, or even physicians and therapists are woefully misinformed or underinformed as to what these disorders are about from a neurological standpoint. I understand the frustration this causes in parents.

When I first started researching neurobehavioral disorders back in the nineties as a parent of a child with ADHD and as a neurology expert, I was very frustrated by the lack of good, accurate information that could explain what was happening in a child's brain. When I asked professionals, I got vague answers about chemical imbalances and genetics and little else. When I read books, I found that they all said the same things. They reviewed the symptoms and then related a number of case histories and examples. They talked about basic treatment with medications. They said these conditions were mostly genetic and couldn't be cured. That was about it. They never clearly stated what the actual problem was and how it produced the symptoms of ADHD, autism, dyslexia, and other disorders. In fact, they were even unclear as to what the actual symptoms of these disorders are.

I began to realize that the lack of real concrete answers was due to the fact that they didn't have real facts as to what these problems are and what is causing them. I could find no single, established neurological theory that was accepted and used in the scientific or educational community. What I did know and could clearly see was that the problem was increasing dramatically. It was obvious to me that whatever we were doing was not working.

Einstein once said the definition of insanity is doing the same thing over and over and expecting a different result. After a while I realized that the reason I was having difficulty finding an answer was because there is not a single answer.

Childhood neurological dysfunctions share many features in common and are often referred to as learning disabilities or behavioral disorders, implying that the primary symptoms affect only classroom behavior and that the rest of development proceeds smoothly and without incident. This is not the case. Each disorder is complex and often involves every system of the body. Science, however, wasn't taking a whole body approach to seeking a solution. It was searching for a solution by focusing on what appeared to be the main issue. With ADHD, it was an attention problem or impulsivity. With dyslexia, it was a reading problem. With autism, it was a socialization and communication problem. No one was looking at the other problems these children had—problems that could help provide clues to the underlying cause. But I did, and I could see that they involve every system in the body, not just the brain. That's how the Brain Balance Program was born.

These disorders may manifest with different symptoms but they are really one and the same problem: a brain imbalance. There is even a name for it—Functional Disconnection Syndrome, meaning areas in the brain, especially the two hemispheres of the brain, are not electrically balanced, or synchronized. This electrical imbalance interferes with the ability of the two hemispheres to share and integrate information, meaning the brain cannot function as a whole. The result is that a child with a brain imbalance has normal or even unusually good skills associated with the higher-functioning area or side of the brain, and unusually bad skills associated with the underactive area or side of the brain. The problem seems to come about because one side of the brain is maturing at a faster rate than the other. As the child develops, this imbalance becomes more significant and the two hemispheres can never fully function as one. The brain is functionally disconnected. Fix the disconnect—that is, get the immature side of the brain to catch up to the other side—and the symptoms go away. So does the disorder.

This is what the Brain Balance Program does and why it is so revolutionary. Most professionals are still approaching and treating these conditions as a single problem, such as attention, learning, socialization, tics, or other symptoms. However, most of these children have a combination of many different symptoms that include sensory, motor, cognitive, academic, emotional, and immune challenges, as well as dietary and digestive symptoms. As I said, they involve basically every system of the body.

The Brain Balance Program addresses all these symptoms by stimulating the slow side of the brain, stimulating it to develop without affecting the other side through a series of sensory-motor and sensory-academic exercises that address the symptoms of the individual child along with dietary, nutritional, and behavioral changes. It gets the two sides to integrate and start working as a whole. There is no other program like it in the world.

Unfortunately, most parents of children with developmental neurobehavioral disorders do not have a good understanding of the nature of their child's dysfunction. They do not understand what is wrong with their children and why they are behaving the way they do. They are also led to believe that there is no solution to the problem. The best fix, they are told, is through medication that will mask the symptoms but not make them go away.

I have been working with children who are labeled with these disorders since 1994 without drugs or other medical interventions and I know *all* symptoms *can* be resolved. ADD, ADHD, dyslexia, and even autism, among others, can become a thing of the past.

Parents and teachers need to know not only that this is possible but that they can make it happen themselves. This is why I wrote this book. *Disconnected Kids* not only offers a clear understanding of what is going on in the brains of children today, but also gives parents and teachers the power to correct it.

Disconnected Kids is based on the same principles of the Brain Balance Program that is being used in Brain Balance Centers in several cities around the country. It is the most comprehensive program available anywhere today. It is the only truly holistic approach to the brain, and the only one that addresses all the symptoms that are troubling these children.

Disconnected Kids is the culmination of my research and what I hope to be the catalyst to stopping this epidemic that is threatening the mental health of children around the world. It is intended to provide a clear understanding as to what is going on inside the brains and bodies of the children who are victims to this new epidemic. It is also intended to empower everyone involved in the lives of these children to do something about it.

I also wanted to write this book in order to help parents who do not have the access or the money to enroll their child in a professionally led course. I want to share what it feels like to see a child who is struggling to learn and be accepted become a happy, well-adjusted, and attentive student with new friends and the promise of a bright future.

There is no more important social issue today. There is no greater problem that threatens the future of our country and our world than what is happening with our children. I have seen this problem coming, and I have created a program that will stop it. I believe that raising awareness through *Disconnected Kids* and giving parents real tools to take immediate action is the quickest way to make an impact now, before it is too late.

PART

1

DISCONNECTED
KIDS

■

1

DIFFERENT SYMPTOMS, ONE PROBLEM

Understanding the Minds of Disconnected Children

■

My teacher asked if anyone in the class ever heard of autism, so I raised my
hand and said, "I have because I used to have autism."
My teacher said, "That can't be because nobody *used* to have autism; you *have*
autism." Then I stood up and explained to everybody
about Brain Balance and how it made my autism go away.

—BECKY, AGE TWELVE

■

A DECADE AGO, you could go a lifetime and never cross paths with a
child with autism. Today, it's rare if you don't know one, or know
someone who knows someone who has an autistic child. Fifty years ago,
a hyperactive and disruptive child was viewed as a "discipline" problem.
Today, attention deficit/hyperactive disorder, commonly called ADHD, is
the most prevalent childhood problem throughout the world. Ten years
ago, most parents had never even heard of Asperger's syndrome, bipolar
disorder, or oppositional defiant disorder. Today it is in the consciousness
of most every parent of a school-age child.

The rise in childhood neurological disorders—mostly described as
behavioral, social, or academic dysfunctions—has risen so sharply that in
2007 the Centers for Disease Control and Prevention called it a "major
health threat." That is putting it mildly. It is, in fact, the most serious threat
to the health and well-being of our children that this country has ever
faced and one that is increasing in epidemic proportions. Consider:

*Autism, which ten years ago was considered a rare disorder, affects 1 out of
every 150 children born.* Just ten years ago, the prevalence of autism was 1
in every 10,000. And it strikes twice as many boys as it does girls. In the

United States, 1 in every 100 newborn baby boys born today will be diagnosed with autism before the age of three. In the United Kingdom, the statistics are even worse: It is estimated that 1 in every 58 children has some form of autism. The rate of autism, however, is the highest among people in California born after 1980.

Other disorders are increasing at the same rate. A 2007 study in Denmark noted, "Recent increases in reported autism diagnoses might not be unique among childhood neuropsychiatric disorders and might be part of a more widespread epidemiologic phenomenon." This study focused on ADHD, Tourette syndrome, and OCD. Other studies have shown similar rates for dyslexia and other learning disabilities.

Last year doctors in the United States wrote an estimated 20 million prescriptions for Ritalin. And this estimate is considered conservative. ADHD is the leading childhood disorder in the world, and Ritalin is the most widely prescribed medication for children. The use of Ritalin increased a staggering 800 percent between 1990 and 1998, even though it has severe side effects and its long-term consequences on the developing mind are still unknown. It is also only effective in less than 70 percent of cases. The drug is becoming so commonplace it is even being prescribed for children as young as age four.

This year, 1.5 million children entering school—that's 1 out of every 6 five- or six- year-olds—will be diagnosed with some type of neurological disorder that affects the ability to learn and socially interact. This is a trend that is expected only to get worse. In the last ten years, the number of children in special education classes in the United States jumped 46.9 percent. In Florida alone, the number of children in special education increased from 6 percent to 13.2 percent—more than double—in just five years.

One in every four children in special education has Tourette syndrome. In fact, doctors believe that this condition, characterized by uncontrolled verbal or muscle tics, is 50 to 75 percent more prevalent than once believed.

These statistics are staggering, to say the least. Yet here is a fact even more disturbing than the epidemic rise in the unhealthy mental state of our children: *The methods that doctors, psychologists, and behavior specialists use to diagnose and treat these conditions have not changed in fifty years.*

What's going on? Or more to the point, what's going wrong? There are, in fact, several things going wrong:

■ The widely held, but erroneous, belief that conditions such as autism, Asperger's syndrome, ADHD, dyslexia, and a host of

other childhood neurological conditions are all separate problems with no acknowledged or explainable root cause, except,
perhaps that many children are genetically predisposed.
- The widely held, but erroneous, belief that there is no cure
possible for these problems.
- The rampant use of psychiatric drugs that mask symptoms but
can't correct these problems, which are, in fact, correctable.
- Well-meaning teachers and other professionals who are using
academic approaches that are actually making these conditions worse and may even be unknowingly contributing to the
soaring statistics.

For the parents of a child with a behavior, social, and/or learning disorder, the diagnosis can be devastating. Typically, parents are told that
there is no known cause for their child's problem—that, most likely, it is
genetic, which makes them feel even worse. But the final blow comes with
the prognosis: *There is no cure.* For some children, parents are told, the
symptoms may subside over the years; but on the other hand, they could
also get worse. At best, the condition can be controlled with
medications—psychiatric drugs, they will eventually learn, with a laun-
dry list of side effects for which long-term consequences are still
unknown.

But psychiatric drugs don't cure the problem; they only disguise the
symptoms. So, parents are advised, talk to the school, talk to your child's
teacher. See a psychologist. Be loving, understanding, and patient. Learn
coping techniques to manage the problem because, they are warned,
neurobehavioral and neuroacademic dysfunctions can get better but they
will never disappear.

But I can tell you that they *can* disappear. They *do* disappear and I
have the fully documented proof on more than 1,000 children to prove
it. It's called the Brain Balance Program, a revolutionary nonmedical
approach that effectively corrects the underlying problem common to
the entire spectrum of seemingly disparate childhood neurological
dysfunctions.

The Brain Balance Program is based on my clinically proven findings that
the way your child's brain functions today is not necessarily the way that it
has to function for the rest of his or her life. My research and the research
of others has found that many children can recover from disorders such as
autism, ADHD, Asperger's syndrome, dyslexia, and others when their

unique developmental needs are met and the underlying causes of these disorders are addressed. Even children with the severest forms of these disorders have the capacity to improve behaviorally and academically and learn skills that will enrich their quality of life.

NEW DISCOVERIES IN BRAIN SCIENCE

Neuroscience has long understood that in order for the human brain to function wholly, large areas of the brain as well as the left and right hemispheres continuously use electrical impulses to communicate. This is essential because each hemisphere performs different functions that allow us to react to the world in which we live. More recent research, however, shows that when the two sides of the brain do not mature at the same rate, the electrical impulses between the two sides get out of balance and interfere with communication. Proof now exists that this communication problem is responsible for a myriad of behavioral, social, and learning difficulties.

Though medicine has traditionally classified these children as having a distinct disorder as defined by a set of symptoms—most notably Autism, ADHD, Asperger's syndrome, and dyslexia, among others—new advances in evaluative capabilities and diagnostic imaging show striking similarities in the brains of children with these conditions. We can now see that virtually all of the conditions that adversely affect behavior and learning are actually related to one problem—an imbalance of electrical activity between areas of the brain, especially the right and the left hemispheres of the brain. There is even a name for it: Functional Disconnection Syndrome (FDS).

FUNCTIONAL DISCONNECTION SYNDROME

The concept of a disconnection syndrome actually dates back to the end of the nineteenth century when scientists became aware that certain neurological conditions are the result of a communication problem between the left and the right hemispheres of the brain rather than an injury to one specific area. They found that this disconnect caused specific symptoms. In 1973, the concept of a functional disconnection was used to explain the symptoms of a condition called *alexia*, which is the inability to read words. A functional disconnect is not the result of an injury to the brain. To me, this said, that if the brain is not injured, then the disconnect can be fixed.

In order for the brain to function normally, the activities in the right and the left hemispheres must work in harmony, much like a concert orchestra. When a certain function can't stay in rhythm, it can throw the entire hemisphere off-key, so the other side tries to tune it out. This can cause disharmony to such a degree that the two sides can no longer effectively share and integrate information. The brain becomes functionally disconnected.

A child with a slow-developing left brain, for example, will have different academic problems and display different behaviors than a child with a slow-developing right brain. He may not be able to read words or be able to stay focused on reading. A child with a right brain dysfunction may not look at you when speaking because the brain's ability to read body language is out of balance. The symptoms are different but the problem is the same—Functional Disconnection Syndrome. There are dozens of other examples, but in its most simplistic explanation, this is why your child does not appear "normal." In fact, when parents first bring this problem to the attention of a doctor or other professional, they often say that their child "seems disconnected." And they are exactly on the mark.

▪ Disconnected Children *Are* Different ▪

CHILDREN with Functional Disconnection Syndrome are different from other children because they *feel* different than other children:

They are disconnected from their bodies. Most children with FDS do not feel their own bodies very well. They have no sense of themselves in space or a sense of feeling grounded. They appear clumsy and uncoordinated and have poor timing and rhythm. They have poor or abnormal muscle tone, which is displayed through poor posture and/or an awkward gait. Their eye movement is not like other children's. They may appear to be gazing into outer space or one eye may lack normal movement (what we call lazy eye).

They are disconnected from their senses. Most children with FDS do not fully experience all five senses—sight, hearing, touch, taste, and smell—

which teach normal children to relate to and interact within the world. Many of these children cannot use more than one sense at a time. When they are forced to use multiple senses together, they become overwhelmed. They become easily distracted by anything they see, hear, or feel, which makes it impossible for them to focus. As a result, they become like slaves to their own environment.

They are socially and emotionally disconnected. Children who can't feel their own body movement cannot intuit the connection between movement and feelings. They can't interpret facial expressions or the tones in a voice that tell them what another person is thinking. Where others express emotion, they may remain stone-faced. This leads to social and emotional disconnection from others, making it very hard or even impossible to develop friendship or relationships with others.

You see, these children seem different from normal children because they *are* different. They are different, because they *feel* different.

Children with FDS don't physically feel the same, or think the same, as other children. They feel disconnected from their bodies and their senses. Some can't feel their bodies at all or don't have a sense of themselves in space. They feel disconnected socially and emotionally.

This disconnect is played out through what you see as unusual or disturbing behavior, ranging from impulsive actions and emotional outbursts to an inability to focus and social isolation.

Children with FDS have many traits in common. They often appear clumsy, have poor muscle tone, and may have an odd habit of tilting the head to one side or another. They may not like to be touched, or may be sensitive to certain sounds or smells. They get sick a lot because their immune systems are out of kilter and most are picky eaters because their digestive systems aren't functioning properly. The individual behavioral symptoms and learning problems that a child displays, however, depend on how the imbalance in the brain is manifesting. Our clinical research during the last ten years has found that, most often, there are three types of disconnect that can result in the symptoms of FDS:

A decrease in electrical activity in areas of either the left or the right hemisphere.

A higher-than-normal level of activity of areas in the higher-functioning (larger) hemisphere.

A combination of decreased activity of areas in the weak (smaller) hemisphere and increased activity of areas in the higher-functioning side.

THE BRAIN *CAN* CHANGE

At one time, scientists believed that the brain cannot change or correct an errant growth pattern. This simply is not the case. Over the last several decades neuroscientists have found that the brain is actually quite plastic, meaning that it has the ability to both physically and chemically change—*if* given the proper stimulation. We have seen through brain imaging scans that, when given the proper stimulation, the weak side of the brain will actually get larger and faster. Spaces between cells will get smaller, and new connections will grow. As a result, the new connections in the weak side of the brain can reconnect with the more mature cells on the functioning side and get back in rhythm. The brain begins functioning again as a whole. Disconnected Children become Reconnected Children.

This is what the Brain Balance Program is all about. It is a revolutionary new way to identify and help children with learning and behavioral disabilities, and it is about to turn conventional thinking on its ear.

▶ *Brain Balance Difference No. 1: The Problem Has a Solution*

Until now, disorders associated with the characteristics that result from a brain imbalance have been considered lifelong problems—without a cure or correction. This simply is not the case. The imbalance can be fixed. The weak areas of the brain can be taught to catch up to the stronger areas, reconnect, and get back into normal syncopated rhythm.

▶ *Brain Balance Difference No. 2: Medications Aren't the Answer*

Until now, the best recourse to control the symptoms has been medications. This simply is not necessary. I am not antimedication; I believe medication is helpful in children with severe symptoms. But medications are not the solution. Brain Balance is a totally holistic, multimodality approach to correcting the imbalance. As the imbalance corrects itself, symptoms diminish and eventually go away. Medication is not required.

▶ *Brain Balance Difference No. 3: Don't Accentuate the Positive!*

Until now, the popular approach to dealing with behavior symptoms in the classroom has been to work on strengthening the strong hemisphere while ignoring the dysfunctional, or "broken," side. This actually makes the problem worse! This approach only makes the higher-functioning side get even stronger while the weakness is ignored. This approach is one of the reasons autism and ADHD are on the rise and why most people believe they cannot be corrected.

Brain Balance does just the opposite—it focuses only on what is "broken." It uses exercises that kick-start growth in the weak hemisphere, so it catches up to the dominant side. I call it the Catch-Up Theory—the brain has the ability to literally catch up with itself to where it should be.

■ Why Your Doctor Didn't Mention FDS ■

YOU'D like to believe that there is a lab test, brain scan, or *something* that physicians, psychologists, and behavioral specialists use to come up with a diagnosis of ADHD, autism, dyslexia, OCD, and the whole roster of childhood neurological disorders. Unfortunately, this is not the case.

There are no consistent anatomic or physical markers for these conditions. A diagnosis of any disorder is purely subjective—based on your answers to a series of questions that relate to your child's symptoms and the way your answers are interpreted. Nothing is concrete except the questions themselves, which come right out of the *Diagnostic and Statistical Manual of Mental Disorders,* which first came out in 1952 and went through its last major revision in 1992. The next major revision is scheduled for 2010 or possibly later.

The DSM-IV, as the 1992 version is called, is universally used by professionals throughout the world to diagnose and classify mental disorders. What is called a "text" version came out in 2000, but it contains only additional information. There have been no revisions, despite the fact that there have been major new findings in the nature of virtually all mental disorders that affect children. There is no mention of Functional Disconnection Syndrome, even though modern research recognizes it as a condition that is opening new doors in understanding and finding a cure for ADHD, autism, and other serious childhood neurological disorders.

If you have a child who has been diagnosed with a neurological behavioral disorder, most likely your doctor or therapist used the DSM-IV to make the call. Here's how getting to a diagnosis usually unfolds:

Through your own concern or, sometimes, at the urging of your child's teacher or even your child's pediatrician, you set up an appointment with a specialist in childhood neurological disorders. After a brief interview with you and your child, the professional agrees that, yes, your child's behavior, social, or academic problem could be a mental impairment. The professional pulls out some disguised, cribbed questionnaire derived from the DSM-IV and asks you about your child's symptoms. The eventual diagnosis is based on the number and length of symptoms that match the criteria for an individual disorder. However, even this process is not as clear-cut as it sounds.

The list of questions that pinpoint symptoms can be vague and, therefore, difficult to answer accurately. And how the professional interprets your answers is, for the most part, subjective. But the worst part is that the final judgment comes from a set of criteria that hasn't changed in sixteen years!

▶ *Brain Balance Difference No. 4: One Problem with One Solution*

Until now, specific symptoms determine the diagnoses of the disorder. Brain Balance, however, considers most learning and behavior disorders as one problem: Functional Disconnection Syndrome. This is why one program—the Brain Balance Program—can be the solution for a seemingly myriad number of conditions.

CONDITIONS THAT CAN BE REVERSED

We have found that the Brain Balance Program can help most children labeled with any learning disability or processing disorder. Brain Balance can also correct the conditions that fall under the cluster of pervasive development disorders, which are characterized by the inability to socialize or communicate normally.

Some researchers believe that more serious neurological disorders, most notably bipolar disorder and schizophrenia, also fall under the umbrella of FDS and, therefore, can be helped through the Brain Balance

Program. While we have not worked with many children with bipolar or schizophrenia in our centers, we believe every child is unique and can benefit from the Brain Balance Program. The conditions that we've had success reversing include:

Attention deficit/hyperactivity disorder (ADHD). The inability to pay attention to the point that it disrupts family, friendships, and the classroom.

Autism and autism spectrum disorders. An extreme inability to communicate normally and develop social relationships often accompanied by behavioral challenges, such as prolonged fixation on an object or group of words, or a complete inability to talk. It is considered the most complex and hardest to understand childhood neurological disorder.

Asperger's syndrome. Similar to autism but with excellent verbal skills. Often referred to as "little professor syndrome" because of high intelligence and an obsessive fixation on specific topics of knowledge.

Childhood disintegrative disorder (CDD). The loss of social and communication skills, but usually more dramatic and developing later than in autism. Can also display significant loss in motor (muscle) skills.

Dyslexia and processing disorders. The inability to discriminate the sounds of letters, which also makes spelling, writing, and speech difficult. It is the most misunderstood of all disorders because it is incorrectly perceived as a reading problem owing to mental reversal or transposition of letters.

Obsessive-compulsive disorder (OCD). An anxiety disorder characterized by a pattern of rituals or obsessive thinking to the point that it interferes with everyday living.

Oppositional defiant disorder (ODD). Characterized by openly hostile and defiant behavior, usually toward authority figures.

Tourette syndrome. Characterized by uncontrollable, sudden, repetitive, and purposeless muscle or verbal tics.

Nonverbal learning disability. Characterized by severely low nonverbal intelligence and average to above average verbal intelligence.

HOW BRAIN BALANCE WORKS

The Brain Balance Program is based on a technique I developed called hemispheric integration therapy (HIT). First, a child is given a series of tests to assess his or her symptoms and functional abilities and determine the hemisphere and functions within the hemisphere that are out of balance. Then a series of daily sensory, physical, and academic exercises are selected that directly target the troubled areas. At first, these exercises are used separately to strengthen functional weaknesses and are then worked simultaneously to integrate large areas of the brain, especially the two hemispheres, and get them back in synchronization. These exercises require about an hour three times a week.

The Brain Balance Program also incorporates a nutritional program to correct dietary problems that are one of the causes of the epidemic rise in childhood neurological disorders. Brain Balance also addresses family-based environmental causes that studies strongly suggest are also linked to the problem.

Our results from the Brain Balance Program have been astounding. Many children with learning difficulties who have gone through my centers have advanced as much as three to eleven grade levels after three months on the program. This is far greater than the results formal private tutoring programs promise in their much-hyped advertisements! We have seen withdrawn children who never spoke become happy, social, academic achievers. You will hear many of their stories throughout this book.

During the last dozen years I have taught more than one thousand health and education professionals around the world how to implement some of the principles of the Brain Balance Program and I am now going to teach you. I believe that the way to stop the epidemic rise in these neurological disorders that are threatening the mental health of future generations is to give as many people as possible the tools to correct these disorders and the information that can help prevent them. To this end, I have adapted my supervised program into one that parents, teachers, and clinicians can use to achieve lasting results. This book is your guide to learning and using the same basic program on your own child at home and achieving measurable, positive results.

As you and your child work your way through the physical, mental, nutritional, and behavioral activities in this book, you should see a gradual change in academic and muscular performance as your child's brain catches up with itself and starts to get into a normal, healthy rhythm. I will lead you all the way to achieving this glorious end. The At-Home Brain Balance Program will show you how to:

- Assess your child for a left or a right brain deficiency.
- Pinpoint the region or regions of decreased electrical brain activity and/or region or regions of accelerated activity.
- Search for nutritional deficits that most likely are contributing to and exacerbating your child's symptoms.
- Make the necessary nutritional changes that will biochemically correct the problem.
- Examine your family lifestyle and home environment and make positive changes.
- Implement behavioral strategies that will help ease family tension—behaviors, by the way, that will eventually go away as the imbalance resolves.

The results you can expect to get are:

- Increased academic performance, even superior grades.
- Decreased negative behavior.
- Elimination of aberrant and/or extreme behavior.
- Marked improvement in communication and social skills.

Before we get started, however, you need a basic understanding of how a child's brain develops and what's happening inside the brain that causes a disconnect.

2

CHILDREN'S BRAINS REALLY *ARE* CHANGEABLE

How the Developing Brain Is Wired

■

When the moment came, Bobby took his place right in
the middle of his peers. There was no meltdown, no crying,
no covering of ears, or shutting of eyes. It was as if autism
left the room and Bobby stayed behind.

—MARILYN, BOBBY'S MOM

■

M OST PEOPLE THINK of brain development as the knowledge we begin stuffing between our ears from the moment we take our first breath. It's not an odd assumption considering that a baby is born with about 100 billion brain cells. That's more brain cells with more connections in one tiny head than there are stars in the galaxy!

You may find this image hard to fathom, especially when you consider that a baby's brain weighs only 12 ounces at birth, about 25 percent of its full size. But there is a logical explanation for this: These brain cells, just like the brain itself, have yet to grow. As they mature, brain cells, called neurons, get larger, stronger, and form tentacle-like branches in order to connect and communicate with other neurons and set the stage for how we will survive and thrive in life—our ability to rationalize, sense the world about us, express emotion, listen, communicate, and learn. This is the true essence of brain development.

. . .

THE BRAIN AT BIRTH

Most people think that we are born with a completely formed brain, just as we are born with all the vital tissue that make the heart beat. This is not so. In fact, the brain is the only organ not fully formed at birth. Only the brain's basic structures are intact. However, the brain starts working as a vital, functioning organ long before it is completely formed.

Brain growth actually starts about 40 days after conception when the cortex, the gray matter that looks like deep wrinkles or grooves, starts to form. The neocortex, as it is called in fetal development, is the seed for the genesis of neurons, which are now sprouting and accumulating rapidly, sometimes at the rate of a quarter million per minute. For the next 125 days, new neurons will continually explode into existence like fireworks from deep within the neocortex. But this will not occur in a haphazard way. Their migration to specific locations will be carefully orchestrated, to a large degree, by genetic code. Some of these neurons will be directed to building the brain itself, forming the six layers that make up the cerebral cortex. By the end of two months, the human cortex in a fetus will be intact and identifiable. Cell migration, however, will continue to flourish, and won't stop until about the end of the fifth month.

Meanwhile, another important aspect of brain development is taking place. Fatty sheaths called glial cells are also sprouting and growing at an even greater speed. Glial cells, or glia, are like the glue of the central nervous system. They are essential to healthy neurons because they spark electrical activity and communication from cell to cell—what scientists call synapses or synaptic connections.

Throughout life, glial cells play an important role in keeping the brain and nervous system active and alive. They are responsible for providing neurons with life-sustaining oxygen and glucose. They assist in the production of axons and dendrites, the tentacle-like structures that are the senders (axons) and receivers (dendrites) of the brain's massive communication system. Glia are also responsible for getting rid of neurons that shrivel up and die. But their main job is powering brain development by forming the neural pathways that govern virtually everything we do, from breathing and learning to thinking and feeling.

Genes are also involved in the production of glia, but only to a limited degree. Growth is mainly dependent on feedback from the mother's body by means of nutrition and stimulation.

After birth, the brain will grow in sequential form from the bottom up—from the brain stem, the least complex area, to the cerebral cortex, the most complex area.

Synapses are now developing at an astounding rate. At birth, few synaptic connections exist—just enough to regulate breathing, heartbeat, blood pressure, metabolism, and other vital functions. During the first year, the average baby will add slightly more tissue to its brain than it will add throughout the rest of its life. By age two, roughly 80 percent of the brain is intact. By age six, the brain is almost 90 percent of its adult size and possesses approximately 1,000 trillion synapses, more than even the smartest person in the world could possibly ever use. This gives the brain virtually limitless processing power.

HOW THE MIND GROWS

Synaptic connections are the key that makes learning—what most people think of as brain development—possible. They are also the key to physical growth, as well. At one time scientists believed that mental and physical growth were mutually exclusive. But this is not the case at all. We now know that one cannot exist without the other. Every biologically important event, from the recognition of a mother's smile or a father's voice to sitting, crawling, walking, and talking are the result of new connections, producing electrical excitement between neurons within the synaptic loop. The Kodak-moment milestones that parents anxiously await are markers of synaptic development and signs of normal neural growth. Even though brain cells accumulate at lightning speed before birth, synaptic connections do not just magically happen. Synapses are dependent on two things for formation and growth: fuel, in the form of oxygen and glucose, and stimulation.

When two neurons are excited together, they become linked functionally. Stimulation reverberates cells, enabling them to continue assembly even after the sensation has ceased. Cell assembly, however, must be repeatedly activated in order to produce synaptic connections. What we now know—and what is at the core of the success of Brain Balance—is that fuel alone will not make brain cells grow; only stimulation does.

As the brain grows in size, it requires more and more fuel to sustain the increasing workload. But all the fuel in the biological universe cannot make cells proliferate in the absence of stimulation. Without stimulation, the brain will not grow. Brain cells will degenerate and die. By age ten, the average child will lose half of the trillion synapses that existed at birth.

You've heard it said: *Use it or lose it.* Well, it doesn't just apply to brains that are getting old and senile. It's essential to making young minds grow.

MAKING HEALTHY BRAINS

Stimulate: *verb; to excite to activity or growth or to greater activity*

This definition from Webster's dictionary is the essence of what brain development is all about. Studies have shown that without proper stimulation, a child's brain suffers. Researchers at Baylor College of Medicine, for example, found that children who don't play much or are rarely touched develop brains 20 to 30 percent smaller than normal. A sad display of what the lack of stimulation can do to the developing brain was classically illustrated several years ago at orphanages in Romania in which abandoned babies, left to lie in cribs without being held, smiled at, or ever hearing a loving coo, experienced underdeveloped brains almost to the point of retardation. These children had stunted brain growth because they were deprived of their sensory world. The senses are the transportation system of mental stimulation. They are the vehicle that drives stimulation to the brain. In fact, the senses and the processes that stimulate the brain are closely entwined.

Although the brain is able to provide a certain amount of stimulation on its own—dreaming is the best example—it is mostly dependent on outside sources to spark neural growth. The outside sources of natural environmental stimuli on which the brain depends are:

Light
Sound or vibration
Odor
Taste
Temperature

Touch
Pressure or gravity

The reflection of sunlight on a beach, the sound of waves crashing to shore, the scent of sea air, the taste of the salty sea, the warmth of a sea breeze, the patter of feet running on the shore, and the movement of playing in the sand can all provoke the senses to stimulate the mind.

The sensory system is equipped with receptors that act like a switch to start the flow of stimulation that activates the brain, much as the flick of a light switch starts the flow of electricity that turns on a lamp. The retina has rods and cones that serve as light receptors. Ears possess cilia, or hair cells, that carry sound. Joints and muscles have receptors that sense movement and gravity. These receptors exist for the sole purpose of collecting information from the environment and sending it to the brain. Like a light switch, these receptors have a set course of circuitry— throughout the nervous system. Stimulation travels the wire from receptors to nerves in the spinal column, then up through the brain stem, and throughout the brain, where it fires a burst of activity in cells. The more a brain cell is stimulated, the more it will increase in size and processing speed, strengthen its connections, and form new synapses. Success is based on three factors:

Frequency of the stimulation
Duration of the stimulation
Intensity of the stimulation

The impulses that stimulate cells most frequently, for the longest period of time, and with the greatest degree of intensity will have the greatest effect on the growth of the cells and the overall speed of brain processing.

Think of a child learning to ride a bicycle. On a three-wheeler a child learns how to steer. He will go round and round in circles until something snaps into place—a new synapse—and he can aim and travel straight down the sidewalk. By repeatedly working on training wheels, a child advances to a two-wheeler and masters the skill of balance. Another example is memorization. Think of the many times you had to read the lines of poetry before you could recite them by heart.

But what is frequency? You're probably already thinking that the kinds of environmental stimuli I am talking about are not constant and are not always available. Light, sound, taste, and temperature are all of variable frequency, duration, and intensity. Sunlight, for example, is only present during the day, and in some parts of the world it is rarely seen at certain times of the year for months on end.

There is, however, one constant source of stimulation from the environment: gravity. We are continually compelled to use our muscles and joints to resist gravity. Because gravity steadily exerts force on us, and because we are perpetually forced to resist it, the amount of time it stimulates the brain based on frequency and duration is much greater than any other sensation. Every movement we make stimulates the brain. Just standing, for example, enables muscles to resist gravity. Repeated muscle activity is the single most important element of brain development. You'll get a greater understanding of this as you go through this book.

TWO SIDES TO EVERY BRAIN

Relative to body size, the human brain is one of the largest among all living species. But it is not just unique in size; it is also unique in structure.

The human brain is so sophisticated and equipped to do so many functions that specific duties reside either on the right or on the left. This means that each side does half the job of the whole. But in order to function, the brain must work as a whole. There is no other brain in the living universe that is built quite this way.

In order for the human brain to function as a whole, the left and right hemispheres must be in constant communication. In order to communicate effectively, the two sides must be able to keep up with each other—they must be in synchronization. They must be in perfect rhythm, perfect harmony, and perfect timing, just like a couple on *Dancing with the Stars*.

In addition to being in sync, the brain's timing mechanism must also be fast enough to keep up with the flow of information. The more the brain develops, the faster the speed gets. The brain must be quick enough to make split-second decisions, like jumping out of the way of a speeding car or ducking to avoid a fly ball. The brain can't perform at such great speed if it is not synchronized.

Consider the rhythmic two-legged control of a world-class athlete running a marathon. As she nears the finish line, she picks up speed, going faster and faster. If one leg suddenly gets a charley horse or trips on a stone, the whole body is crippled because one leg can't keep up with the other. They get out of sync. The good leg can get her to the finish line, but she'll fall behind the pack. And the farther away she is from the finish, the farther behind she will get from the others.

This, in essence, is what is happening in school to a child with Functional Disconnection Syndrome. The brain's in-sync timing mechanism is the foundation of all thinking, movement, behavior, sensory response, and vital functions, such as breathing and digestion. Each half of the brain contributes differently to our understanding of and our reactions to the world in which we live. Each side of the brain responds differently to stimulation. Sensory experiences are also processed differently in the two hemispheres.

To fully understand the world and react to it, a child must use both sides of the brain as a whole. If one half of the brain is significantly slower than the other, the two halves cannot compare or share information accurately. When one side of the brain is too slow, the faster, or stronger, side takes over and begins to ignore the other, underactive side. When this happens, a child's interpretation of and reactions to the world around him will be "off," so to speak, and his behavior will appear abnormal.

This is what I believe is the primary problem in Disconnected Children. Children have learning and behavioral dysfunctions because their brains are out of sync. I believe it is responsible for many if not all of the physical, mental, and/or behavioral and social difficulties related to the whole spectrum of childhood neurological disorders.

THE BRAIN CAN CHANGE

Conventional medical wisdom long held the belief that the human brain cannot change—that it is hardwired at birth just like a computer. Scientists started to collect evidence in the early 1970s that eventually proved this is not the case. They found that the brain is actually malleable and has the ability to change both physically and chemically in response to certain types of activity. They found that it can change its shape, size, number of branches, number of connections, as well as the strength of its connections.

The potential of this ability is so far reaching, it has become a science of its own called neuroplasticity—*neuro* meaning neurons and *plastic* meaning changeable.

■ Albert Einstein's Learning Disability ■

ALBERT Einstein, the Nobel Prize–winning Father of Relativity, is considered one of the greatest minds of all time, but as a child he was far from brilliant. In fact, scientists now agree that Einstein had a significant learning disorder that today would be diagnosed as ADHD and/or dyslexia.

He did not speak until he was around age seven and did poorly academically all the way through college. When he failed to get into graduate school at the age of twenty, he became a clerk in the Swiss Patent Office. But he did not give up his cerebral pursuits. Just six years later he published the first draft of his scientific Theory of Relativity, which won him the Nobel Prize ten years later.

So, what can turn the mind of a child who can't pass the grade into a veritable, well, Einstein? The answer is neuroplasticity, the brain's ability to change and grow. When Einstein's brain was examined after he died in 1955, it appeared basically the same as everyone else's. It was roughly the same size and shape as most brains and had the average number of brain cells. One scientist, however, discovered something uniquely different about Einstein's brain: It possessed an enormous number of connections, or synapses, between brain cells. While at one time this could have been credited to good genes, we can now see that a great deal of Einstein's genius was the result of the unique way he used his brain.

Einstein was passionate about music and played the piano and violin regularly. When he was stuck on a mathematical problem, he once explained, he would sit down and play music and envision his problem until the mathematical equation came to him. Put another way, listening to music (the sense of hearing) stimulated playing an instrument (physical activity), which is a right brain activity, and concentration on the equation (mental activity), which is a left brain activity. Doing so on a repetitive basis not only strengthened the electrical connections (communication) between the cells in the left and right hemispheres of Einstein's brain, but also caused new connections to grow. Combined, they increased his brainpower. He became a genius.

> The same thing can happen to your child. The Brain Balance Program combines physical exercise and mental exercise with sensory stimulation to get the left and right sides of the brain to reconnect, strengthen, and grow new connections. When this happens, the behavior problems created by the brain imbalance and the nutritional problems that contributed to the problem start to disappear. ■

At birth, the brain has merely developed the blueprint of what it is yet to be. Neural activity, driven by a flood of sensory experiences, will direct brain growth and progressively refine it. As a baby grows into a toddler and then a school-age child, she will become more dependent on the environment for the stimulation that will drive the development of the cerebral cortex, the largest and most complex part of the brain that molds the way a child will think, act, and achieve. A brain may be genetically wired for greatness, but neural activity within this region is what will eventually determine if it will come to fruition. These are the facts and findings that led me to suspect that the alarming rise in conditions such as autism, ADHD, and dyslexia has more to do with the environment than genetics.

These facts and findings also have profound positive implications for a child with Functional Disconnection Syndrome because they are proof that a child's brain can be rewired. When given the right stimulation for the right amount of time that is directed to the right place in the brain, an imbalance between the two hemispheres of the brain can be fixed.

In the past, doctors and therapists have used therapies that stimulate the whole brain. But they haven't been effective because stimulating both sides doesn't work well. In fact, it can make the imbalance worse. The Brain Balance Program is so effective because it stimulates only the weak side of the brain, so it can strengthen and grow without interfering with the stronger, faster side. It is not so difficult that parents cannot do it themselves. But before I teach you how to identify an imbalance in your child and show you how to correct it, you first need to understand what happens to a child when the left and the right brain get out of sync.

■ How Brain Cells Work ■

A BRAIN cell has but two jobs: It receives and transmits information. That's it. But it is an awesome responsibility because it is this process, which is continually taking place among millions of cells, that makes the brain function.

Brain cells receive and transmit information through electrical impulses that are transmitted mostly through the release of certain chemicals known as neurotransmitters. The information enters the body through stimulation from the environment and travels to the brain on receptors in the form of light, sound, smell, taste, temperature, and touch. Larger receptors send signals to larger brain cells, and smaller receptors send signals to smaller brain cells. Most large cells send their signals to the right brain, and smaller cells send their signals to the left brain.

When environmental stimuli hit the receptor, it is like pressing a button. A small amount of stimulus presses the button slowly; a lot of stimulus presses the button very fast. The speed or frequency of pressing the buttons is dependent on the amount of stimulation in the environment.

3

WHEN THE BRAIN MISBEHAVES

A Left Brain, Right Brain Disconnect

■

I hardly realized that I had a body except
when I was hungry or when I realized that I was standing
under the shower and my body got wet ... Every movement is a proof that I
exist. I exist because I can move.

—TITO, AGE THIRTEEN

■

A N INFANT ENTERS the world with just enough brainpower to keep the heart beating, the lungs breathing, the bowels moving, and other less obvious necessities that support life.

An infant, for example, can't see very well. When a mother holds her newborn for that first face-to-face introduction, she may be looking at the most beautiful being on earth but her baby is gazing at a muted, gray image. He can hear and respond to Mother's voice but high-frequency sound is yet to tune in. Baby can't move his head, eyes, or those little fingers and toes either. But not for long. The sensory overload that fires the neural synapses that turn on the color and tune in the world is already picking up speed. The world itself is now the major source of sensory stimulation.

A TIME MACHINE

Among the many complexities of the human brain is its timing mechanism. Though the brain is reliant on left and right brain balance to function normally, it doesn't grow in a balanced way. In the womb and during the first few years of life, brain growth is focused almost exclusively on the right hemisphere, the big picture window to the world. The right brain drives big muscle tasks. For instance, it allows a baby to move her little arms and legs and turn her head. The left brain is growing, too, but not as actively. This is a crucial time in brain development and is the foundation on which all future skills will be built.

Around age two, growth switches mostly to the left brain, the center of small picture thinking, or what we call local processing. This is the center where those first words form. From then on, development switches back and forth between left and right until about the age of ten, when the brain reaches its adult size.

Another complexity of the human brain is its asymmetry (what scientists call lateralization). The processes that allow a child to think, move, express emotion, and interact socially reside in either the right or the left hemisphere of the brain. In other living species, brain centers are stored on both sides. Asymmetry is what enables the human brain to package all of its power.

WHY MILESTONES ARE IMPORTANT

Scientists have yet to isolate what happens to throw brain growth out of kilter to the point that it leads to future difficulties in thinking and behaving, but there is evidence that it has a lot to do with the brain's sensitive timing mechanism during development.

We know, for instance, that sensory stimulation and activity are not random. The senses pick up stimulation and lead it to the brain in a very methodical way to create specific parts of the brain. This is why those childhood milestones are so important—so don't let your child's pediatrician tell you otherwise. One new skill leads to another new skill and it is supposed to happen at an expected point in time. When it doesn't, it is a warning flag.

■ The Skewed Wiring of Autism ■

AUTISM is the most extreme on the continuum of disorders that I collectively call Functional Disconnection Syndrome.

Autistic children appear healthy but act abnormally. They may stare into space for hours or become fixated on a spot on the floor that others don't even notice. They may act out and frequently throw tantrums. They are also antisocial. They show no interest in people, and may engage in peculiar activities, such as hand flapping.

New research into this baffling condition has given scientists important details as to how autism develops. Trained specialists in childhood development have found that the brains and heads of autistic children develop in similar out-of-sync patterns.

Using a simple tape measure, researchers at the University of California, San Diego, found that newborns who later develop autism have smaller head circumferences than average. During the first month of life, the brain suddenly begins to grow rapidly and the head grows much too fast. Another growth spurt occurs between six months and two years, giving rise to exceptionally large heads. Brain growth gradually slows from ages two to four, reaching a peak a year later. A five-year-old autistic child can have the same size brain as a normal thirteen-year-old but by midadolescence, when normally developing children catch up, an autistic child's brain is again comparatively smaller. Moreover, the areas of the brain that show excessive growth also show signs of chronic inflammation.

Ruth Carper, PhD, of the University of California, San Diego, found that the frontal lobes, the slowest and last brain region to develop, have the biggest size increase of all. But the nerve cells in this region are actually much smaller than normal, meaning they are underpowered. This provides important clues into the manner in which autism manifests because the frontal lobes are responsible for high-level functioning, including social reasoning and decision making.

Other research has found that subtle abnormalities in brain circuitry are present even at birth. Imaging tests show that some parts of the autistic brain have too many connections while other parts have too few. Using a new postmortem technique called morphometric analysis, Martha Herbert, MD, a pediatric neurologist at Harvard Medical School, found an anomaly in the white matter of autistic brains—it is asymmetrical. In autism, white matter grows normally until nine months. Then it goes haywire. By age two years, excessive white matter is found in the frontal lobes, the cerebellum, and other areas where high-order processing occurs.

Research from the laboratory of Marcel Just, DO, a neuroscientist at Carnegie Mellon University, reaffirms the odd circuitry in autism. He found that children with autism remember letters of the alphabet in a part of the brain that ordinarily processes shapes. Skewed brain wiring helps explain why autistic children are often clumsy. ▪

Milestones are the obvious checkpoints that brain development is not going according to nature's schedule. This happens when the electrical activity that generates brain growth gets out of timing. There are millions of electrical actions taking place within the brain at any given moment that keep currents flowing like a rushing river. If a child isn't exposed to the proper stimulation at the right time, or if a sensory pathway is too weak, neurons destined to build a new site and set a new milestone miss their time to connect. When this happens too frequently, or during a critical part of brain development, the brain's growth pattern can get out of sequence and cause a slowdown in a key growth area. This causes the side of the brain that missed the connection to slow down as well. Meanwhile, the opposite side stays on track, leaving the other behind. This can cause the other side to miss even more timed connections.

Most often, this occurs during the most crucial times of right brain development—before birth and during the first two years of life. But this only becomes apparent later on when the child starts to exhibit the symptoms we see as ADHD, autism, dyslexia, and other neurological disorders. Some of these symptoms can be evident even in infancy. These symptoms differ according to when the delay in development occurred, but the result is one and the same: Functional Disconnection Syndrome. Symptoms are the clues that tell us if the delay occurred in the left brain or the right brain. Here are those symptoms.

POOR BODY AWARENESS

Poor spatial orientation, or proprioception, is the quintessential definition of Disconnected Children—they simply don't know where they are in space. They don't feel grounded. It is very possible that some children with FDS haven't been able to feel their bodies very well from the time they were born.

Unfortunately, most children can't tell us that they feel this way. However, *you* can tell by observing the way they move their bodies. Here's how to look for these signs:

Children who can't feel themselves in space have a poor sense of gravity and, as a result, are not very good with balance. They are clumsy and will walk into things. With eyes closed while standing, they wobble and stagger. If you ask them to close their eyes and put their feet together, they will fall to the side.

Some children, particularly those diagnosed with ADHD, don't pay attention to all the space around them. They ignore what's happening to their left and may even appear to drag their left side. We've found that they even will visually miss the left half of words, which, obviously, hinders their reading ability.

▪ Proprioception: You Can't Live Without It ▪

A CHILD can adapt and function normally without the sense of sight or sound, but will struggle even with just a weak sense of proprioception.

Proprioception, often referred to as the sixth sense, is the ability to use muscle control and balance to resist gravity. It is also the greatest sensory stimulus for brain growth because, unlike all other sensory stimulation, it occurs 24/7.

Children with Functional Disconnection Syndrome are usually physically awkward. They may walk oddly, be unusually clumsy, lean to one side, or be unable to get the hang of riding a bicycle. This is because they don't feel their bodies very well. Some can't even feel their bodies at all; they don't have a sense of themselves in space. This is a sign of a proprioception problem.

Gravity is such a strong stimulus that life cannot survive very long without it. When scientists sent organisms into outer space to test the lack of gravity on the brain, they found rapid and significant degeneration of brain cells. NASA coined the phrase "space dyslexia" for astronauts who came back from space missions with mental processing problems similar to children with diagnosed learning disabilities.

We resist gravity by using our large muscles and joints. And it is an important function to have. In one study, scientists at the University of California at Berkeley found that when rats used their muscles and joints in new and interesting ways, they showed increased plasticity and growth in their brain. When sent into space, the same kind of rats showed reverse plasticity and a rapid degeneration of brain cells.

It takes only a small leap to recognize that a child who is sitting in front

of the television or computer for hours at a time is not maximizing his or
her use of gravity as a stimulus to brain development.   ■

These children seem to lack a kind of internal map that normal children develop in their first few years. Many cannot identify parts of their bodies in a mirror. Even if they know they have a nose, when asked to point to it, they'll put a finger on, say, an ear instead.

Feeling physically disconnected has a profound effect on a child's ability to develop emotionally and socially. Children who do not feel gravity do not feel safe and grounded and are not able to form normal emotional relationships even with their families. Mothers often tell me that this disconnect was the first clue that something was wrong with their child. This lack of self-image is also at the root of another prominent symptom: poor socialization.

POOR GROSS AND FINE MOTOR SKILLS

All children with FDS share one major trait: They have problems with motor skills—their muscles do not move fluidly.

Virtually all these children were delayed and have difficulty learning how to use their large muscles, what we call gross motor skills. As a result, they usually have poor muscle tone throughout the body. Most noticeable is bad posture and an awkward gait. They are uncoordinated and have no sense of timing or rhythm.

Children with FDS are often very late in reaching early motor milestones, particularly crawling and walking. They may crawl in an unusual pattern, such as scooting on their bottoms. Many skip crawling altogether and start walking earlier than usual. Most, however, start walking late, and may appear unsteady or fall. While seated, they may fall over to the side if unsupported. This is due in part to a delay in developing the muscles in the back and near the spine that support normal posture.

These children often have motor symptoms so subtle that they often go undetected. A head tilt or a body tilt to one direction, for example, is a sign that postural muscles are out of balance. A foot that turns in and legs that appear knock-kneed are other signs of improper postural muscle growth and tone.

Children with FDS also often have trouble manipulating their hands, fingers, toes, and feet—what we call fine motor skills. This most often is displayed later on as poor handwriting.

PERSISTENCE OF PRIMITIVE MOTOR REFLEXES

While in the womb and during the first weeks of life, a baby can move only essential muscles—the trunk, head, mouth, and eyes. He can move his arms and legs but with very little control. These are what we call primitive reflex movements.

A baby's instinctive head turn to suckle is the most obvious primitive reflex that a parent will notice. Another is the way a baby flexes when she turns her head. When the head turns in one direction, the arm and leg on the same side will straighten out as the other arm and leg flex. Babies are supposed to outgrow their primitive reflexes as the stronger postural muscles start to form. They should be gone by the end of the first year. However, in some children they linger longer. This can throw off the timing for the development of the large muscles and is an early symptom of problems to come.

Problems performing primitive motor reflexes, such as difficulty suckling or an inability to feed at the breast, are also a sign of improper brain development.

▪ Left-Handed, Right-Footed ▪

WE HAVE two feet, two hands, two eyes, two ears, and even two brains. Left and right—the perfectly symmetrical human form. But human symmetry is literally in the eye of the beholder. When it comes to function, we are decidedly one-sided.

The most obvious, of course, is handedness. By about the age of two, it should be obvious if your child favors his left or right hand. But did you know that your child also has a dominant foot, ear, and eye as well?

Most people, some 90 percent of the population, are right-handed. It is not uncommon for a child with FDS to be left-handed, but this in itself is not cause for alarm. It is not handedness but what we call mixed dominance, or cross-laterality, that raises the red flag.

Optimally, hand, foot, eye, and ear dominance should all be on the same side of the body. In most people this is the right side. This is believed to take advantage of left brain control of language and voluntary motor skills. A much larger percentage of children with learning disabilities and behavioral disorders have mixed dominance. They may be right-handed, left-footed, right-eyed, and left-eared. This is a deviation from normal because it slows brain speed. Think about it: If the dominant eye and the ear are on opposite sides, vision circuits have to jump to the other side of the brain to connect to the listening circuits. This may take but a fraction of a second, but this is slow to the brain's lightning speed and can interfere with a child's ability to keep up in school. It is a common reason why some people can't read and listen at the same time.

A mixed-dominance profile, by the way, has been shown to be higher in children who have had stressful births.

POOR EYE COORDINATION

Children may often have a slight imbalance in the tone of the eye muscles. This can appear as lazy eye, in which one eye turns out or doesn't move with the other. Another sign is an inability to cross the eyes well.

A less obvious sign is poor eye coordination in which both eyes cannot easily track a moving object. One or both may overshoot or undershoot a target when tracking quickly. This contributes to reading difficulties.

POOR SOCIAL SKILLS

Poor social skills are not only a very common symptom of FDS, they are a significant problem. Sadly, most of these children are very friendly and motivated to have social relationships but they don't know how to go about it. They do it all wrong.

Normal development of social skills is dependent on the normal development of the area of the brain that controls nonverbal communication. Nonverbal communication is the ability to read body language—that is, understanding people's emotions and intentions by observing their body posture, facial expression, tone of voice, and the like. This is not a skill that can be taught; it develops naturally and subconsciously during brain development early in life. In fact, new research tells us it may begin as early as three months of age. If a child's brain is too slow in developing nonverbal communication skills, it will affect his or her ability to "read" people and relate to them socially.

■ Why "Talking" Doesn't Work ■

PRACTITIONERS and parents make a mistake in dealing with children with autism, Asperger's, and ADHD who speak very little or not at all. They focus on trying to make them talk because they fail to understand that the real problem is not with verbal communication, but with nonverbal communication.

Verbal communication cannot happen unless nonverbal communication is learned first.

Nonverbal communication is the foundation of verbal communication. It develops first. So if nonverbal skills don't develop properly, a child will be delayed or unable to communicate verbally: Without the ability to communicate, a child can't develop social skills.

This is also why it is almost impossible to teach socialization skills. Children who go through socialization training may learn the rules of social interaction but they never really learn how to socialize normally. Socialization cannot be consciously learned because it is a subconscious skill that must develop naturally. ■

ABNORMAL EMOTIONAL REACTIONS

A child who is slow in developing nonverbal skills will also have problems developing emotionally for the same reasons.

Emotional and social development is orchestrated by a special network of brain cells called mirror neurons. They subconsciously communicate the emotion of what we see and hear. Mirror neurons drive the nonverbal communication system that relays laughter and a smile as happiness and crying and a frown as disappointment. It is why we can distinguish a scream coming from another room as one of joy or one of fright.

When a baby sees facial expressions and body postures in others, mirror neurons trigger and simulate the same internal chemical responses and instinctive movements of their muscles to mirror the same emotions. The brain says, "I know what that person is feeling because I feel the same way when I move my body that way." The image is then imprinted in the brain. The child can get "in touch" with others' emotions as well.

When Mom smiles and baby smiles back, it means mirror neurons are on the job. At least, this is the way it is supposed to happen.

A child who cannot feel her own body and is not adept at nonverbal communication, however, lacks the skills that distinguish a scream of joy from a scream of fright. At best, she will struggle making friends and interacting with others. At the worst, she will simply have no ability to understand emotional expression. As a result, she will act in socially unacceptable ways.

SENSORY PROCESSING SYMPTOMS

I have yet to see a child with Functional Disconnection Syndrome who does not have an abnormally sensitive sensory system. A fussy eater has an undersensitive sense of taste and smell. Some children cover their ears because they can't stand a noise that sounds normal to everybody else. Some don't like to be hugged, even by their parents.

There is usually something amiss with at least one of the senses—taste, smell, sight, hearing, and touch—in children with FDS. A child's sensitivity could involve one or more than one sense; it could even involve all the senses. It could be that one of the senses is supercharged and another is undercharged. Some children with FDS may even have diagnosed sensory integration disorder, meaning that the entire sensory system is substandard in supplying the brain with stimulation. It is pretty much a given that when the brain's timing is off in processing one sense, the others will suffer. It is common for a child to struggle when trying to use several senses at the same time.

A healthy sensory system is essential to healthy brain development because it is the solo driver of stimulation to the brain. Each sense plays an important role in the journey. When they're all well tuned, they'll send signals to the brain like a bullet train. But the ones that get off track can slow down the process and make the journey travel like the local train.

A deficit in one or more of the senses causes what we call a processing disorder. However, I see it as an important symptom causing Functional

Disconnection Syndrome. How the senses are affected is key in identifying whether the imbalance is in the left or the right hemisphere of the brain. These are the symptoms you'll be looking for.

▶ *Vision*

I like to illustrate a visual processing problem with these questions: Do you see something? What do you see? In other words, can you see the forest for the trees?

A child with a visual processing problem literally has trouble detecting the forest for the trees. In fact, optometrists have found that many children with learning disabilities have normal 20/20 eyesight but reduced fields of vision. Some of these children can even have large blind spots in their field of vision. This is a sign that they are having difficulty processing light. As a result, they will be either oversensitive or undersensitive to light.

A visual sensory problem has a direct influence on a child's ability to learn because the part of the brain responsible for processing light is slow. As a result, the brain is slow at processing what the child is seeing.

The visual sensory system consists of two pathways, each with a specific job. One is referred to as the "what" system and the other is the "where" system.

The where system, located in the back of the brain, turns on the big picture. It is responsible for peripheral vision and helps the brain detect motion. It locates objects in space. However, it does not see color. The what system, located in front of the brain, focuses on the small picture. It picks up details and turns on the color. It also detects motion but is slower at processing it.

What we are finding is that children with learning disabilities can't see the forest for the trees because they cannot process visual information properly. In other words, their brains have difficulty blending together the big and small pictures.

In many instances, a child will be very good at small picture skills and very poor at big picture skills. They may actually become poor at one skill because they are so good at the other. The imbalance gets tipped too often in one direction! These children often start out as early readers, some as early as eighteen months.

Without normal visual processing ability, a child cannot put information together and extract higher-level meaning. We call this weak central coherence. Many children with FDS, for example, can read a story but they can't understand what it is all about.

This inability is obvious in children diagnosed with autism and Asperger's. They may excel at remembering details, numbers, sequences, and important dates; they may be able to recall the exact words to a story; but they can't explain what it's all about. In dyslexia, it is just the opposite.

▶ Hearing

Like vision, the brain processes hearing on two levels. There is a basic processing system and a high-level processing system. The basic system is the auditory equivalent of the where system in vision. It is most interested in localizing sounds in space. It is also more tuned to listen for the emotional tone of the person speaking. It does not focus on words and hears more lower-pitched sounds.

The high-level system is the auditory equivalent of the what system. It is more tuned to the details of what is being said. It hears higher-pitched sounds that change rapidly, like the sounds of letters forming a word. Also like vision, it is not unusual for a child with an auditory processing deficit to test normal on a hearing test.

■ A Sound *and* Light Problem ■

IT IS not uncommon for a child with FDS to have a problem processing both hearing and vision.

Researchers discovered this in a fun experiment for kids—a sound and light test. In the test, a clap of sound quickly follows a flash of light. Researchers found that children with normal sensory perception can correctly tell which came first, the sound or the light within just a few milliseconds. Children with hearing processing deficits reported that the sound and light occurred at the same time unless they were 2 to 3 seconds apart!

All the children who detected the sound and light incorrectly had diagnoses of either autism, ADHD, or dyslexia, conditions on the continuum collectively known as Functional Disconnection Syndrome. It's another piece of the proof that these individual conditions are actually one and the same. ■

A hearing processing problem can manifest as either a high-frequency or a low-frequency insensitivity. A child with a high-frequency insensitivity, for instance, will have a problem hearing the sounds of words. This is known as phonological awareness and it is believed to be one of the main causes of dyslexia. Children who cannot hear all the sounds and all the words cannot read the words.

A child with a low-frequency insensitivity will have trouble hearing the inflection in someone's voice that conveys emotion. This is known as prosody and children who can't hear this will have difficulty with non-verbal communication and socialization. A child may be particularly good at hearing high-frequency sounds and poor at hearing lower frequencies, which is characteristic in autism, or just the opposite, which is a main contributor to dyslexia.

Some children can have such sensitive hearing that they are constantly covering their ears because they can't stand the noise. Some are so sensitive that they will obsessively make high-pitched noises.

Temple Grandin, PhD, a college professor who was diagnosed with high-functioning autism syndrome, has written several books about her struggles growing up. "My hearing is like having a hearing aid with the volume control stuck on 'super loud,'" she wrote. "It is like an open microphone that picks up everything. I have two choices: turn the mike on and get deluged with sound, or shut it off. Mother reported that sometimes I acted like I was deaf."

Ears pick up sound from the environment and send it over the airwaves via hairy receptor cells called cilia to the middle ear and the brain, which interprets the sound and sends it back out as the sound you will hear. If the auditory system is out of sync, the sound it is picking up will be off and the brain will not be able to re-create it correctly. What is being said may actually not be what a child is hearing. If a child has a problem modulating sound, for example, he may not be able to discern the inflection in someone's voice. A voice expressing excitement can come across as a monotone. This is another problem that can contribute to a child's inept social skills.

Some children can have a problem processing sounds that change rapidly. For example, they may not be able to detect a difference in the sounds *ba* and *da,* which are only different in the first few milliseconds. This means that they can totally miss syllables in a word or words in a sentence. This is really the essence of the reading problem that is the hallmark of dyslexia.

One of the most extraordinary examples of a skewed auditory system is found in children diagnosed with autism. Some autistic children have been known to have perfect pitch, which is a rare gift in the general population. They can exactly recognize a musical note by the single tap of a key. If an entire song is played, however, they may not recognize it at all.

▶ Touch

A sensitivity to touch can be disarming to parents, especially if they don't understand what is motivating the behavior.

Some children with FDS can be extremely sensitive to touch. They'll squirm away from a hug and keep a distance when sitting with their family. Others are undersensitive and may be overly clinging and constantly want to lean on you. They crave touch. It is almost like feeling numb.

At the opposite extreme are children who do not feel pain very well. An autistic child, for example, can bang and bang his head against the ground without any pain reaction.

Touch-sensitive children frequently will dislike light touch—brushing their hair, for instance—but will be soothed by deep touch, such as scrubbing the scalp. Parents often tell me that their child was unusually good as a toddler and never went through the infamous terrible twos. They say their child was easygoing and didn't complain a lot. They'll go on to say that their child's behavior changed and became quite unruly at the age of six or so. This immediately sends me the clue that their child was delayed in developing a tactile sensory system. Terrible twos behavior is actually normal. It is a good thing. It says that a child is starting to get in touch with her own body. Children explore because they want to connect. This is when they start to form their likes and dislikes. It is an important milestone in brain development.

▶ Smell and Taste

Most parents complain that their kids are fussy eaters. And most kids *are* fussy eaters. You're not going to find any three-year-old asking for herring and sour cream for lunch.

Kids typically have a limited menu of foods they will eat because they have yet to refine their sense of smell and taste. Some kids, however, don't like even popular kinds of foods. This is a sign of a brain imbalance.

I have found in my own clinical experience that a significant number of children with neurobehavioral disorders have a poorly developed or completely absent sense of smell. When tested, many of these children do not even know how to sniff. They will blow out of their nose instead of breathing in. They can't even do it after being shown how. This surely says that they do not smell well.

The sense of smell is one of our most basic senses. Research shows that it is also very important to the ability to learn, memorize, and socialize.

Children who do not smell and taste very well judge food not by taste but rather by how it feels in their mouths. They may avoid cookies simply because they don't like the mouth feel. Normally developing kids, on the other hand, learn to ignore how food feels and are driven solely by taste and smell, especially if it is sweet.

This is significant because this is the same area of the brain that helps drive goal-directed behavior—not only in food choices but in the social realm as well. An area known as the right frontal insula cortex may, in fact, be the link that explains all of the unusual behaviors seen in autism and other neurobehavioral disorders. Smell and taste, emotional touch, nonverbal communication, immune suppression, gut regulation and digestion, intuition, "gut feelings" and subconscious body awareness, vestibular and spatial sense, mirror neuron function and nonverbal communication, and emotional awareness in self and others all converge in this area of the brain. Therefore, a decrease in the sense of smell and taste may have a much greater significance than its effect on eating and food choices.

COMPROMISED IMMUNE SYSTEM

The brain is the controller of the immune response; it's not the other way around. The immune system is a great example of how the two hemispheres of the brain work together as a whole. As with most bodily operations, the immune system resides in both sides of the brain but each hemisphere has a distinct job. The left immune center is like the National Guard. It activates antibodies when illness threatens. The right side suppresses the immune system by preventing it from becoming overactive—kind of like making sure the National Guard keeps the peace without starting a war. However, when the immune system does wage war, it sometimes attacks itself. Havoc erupts in the form of autoimmune diseases, like allergies and asthma.

So, in a left brain deficiency, immune defenses will be down. Bacteria, viruses, and other enemies get to cross the line of least resistance and head for the sinuses, lungs, respiratory system, or wherever else they want to set up residence. Kids with left brain deficiencies get sick a lot. If something is going around, they always catch it. They get lots of ear infections and it is not unusual for them to have had fifteen to twenty rounds of antibiotics by the time they are eight or nine years old.

A right brain deficiency puts the immune system in overdrive. It goes to the defense, even in the absence of an enemy, and speeds out of control. In addition to asthma and allergies, it can create more subtle problems in the form of chronic food sensitivities.

A child with FDS more than likely has an immune system that is out of whack. It is either overactive or underactive. Either way it shows up as a child who gets sicker significantly more than normal. It is a predominate feature in children with FDS.

These are the kids who always catch the cold or whatever infections are going around. They end up with chronic ear infections. They tend to have lots of allergies.

Many of these children have extremely weak immune responses and suffer from chronic infections. Others seem to have overactive immune systems that lead to autoimmune problems like eczema, asthma, and allergies. Often, though, these immune responses are more subtle and show up as chronic inflammation or food sensitivities rather than food allergies.

In fact, many consider autism an autoimmune disorder that leads to chronic lifelong inflammation not only of the body but of the brain as well.

Only it is not. These immune symptoms are not the cause of neurological disorders. Rather, like the other symptoms discussed here, they are part of the greater problem. They are also the key to the solution, which is why the next chapter is devoted to this subject.

RAPID HEARTBEAT AND IMMATURE DIGESTION

A child is born with a primitive nervous system that controls automatic life functions, such as breathing, heartbeat, and digestion. This is called the limbic system—what animals have as their primary brain.

The limbic system also provides the basic survival skills for hunger, thirst, and protection. A baby reacts very impulsively based on his immediate survival needs. This is why babies cry and scream when they need something or they feel threatened or frightened.

As a child's brain grows and matures, the higher centers take over control of these automatic body functions. This usually kicks in around the age of three. The bigger cortex then inhibits, slows down, and improves the function of the heart and digestive system.

When there is a delay in the development of this important part of the brain, a child will continue to have a rapid heartbeat, shallow breathing, and immature digestion. These symptoms are often confusing to pediatricians because a child will appear otherwise healthy.

FOOD SENSITIVITIES

The food sensitivities that plague children with FDS are not the food allergies that many parents are familiar with. There is a big difference between the two. For one, it usually isn't hard to figure out if your child has a food allergy. Symptoms will show up immediately or in a few hours as hives, watery eyes, sneezing, or difficult breathing. It can even result in life-threatening anaphylactic shock. This is the kind of allergy in which a child eats a peanut and almost dies. This is the kind of allergy most parents are familiar with and cautious about. Only about 10 percent of children with FDS, however, have this type of allergy.

Some 85 percent of children with FDS have food sensitivities. They do not produce an allergic reaction that results in physical symptoms; rather, they produce an inflammatory response that results in more subtle mental and behavioral symptoms that can take anywhere from six to seventy-two hours to appear. Research confirms that there is a direct correlation between this type of food sensitivity and an imbalance in the brain.

When parents bring their children to one of my Brain Balance Centers for an evaluation, one of the questions we ask is: *Does your child have any food allergies or sensitivities?* Most answer *no* and will argue that they'd know if their child had a bad reaction to a certain food. Then I explain why they are mistaken.

Unlike the obvious and often frightening physical symptoms of allergies, food sensitivities are hard to identify without a blood test because the symptoms appear gradually. These symptoms include but are not limited to:

Irritability and occasional meltdowns
Inability to focus or concentrate
Impulsive actions
Aggressive behavior
Fatigue
Bedwetting
Sleep disturbances, such as bad dreams and frequent awakening
Learning disabilities
Hyperactivity

A child can be sensitive to almost any food, but the most common sensitivities are to gluten, a proteinlike substance found in wheat products, and casein, a protein found in milk products. Gluten and/or casein are found in pasta, pizza, bagels, milk, cereal, and macaroni and cheese.

Other foods that commonly cause sensitivities include:

Chocolate
Citrus fruit—oranges, grapefruits, lemons, etc.
Corn
Eggs
Legumes—peas, beans, peanuts, and soy
Sugar
Tomato
Yeast products

POOR DIGESTION

If any area of a child's brain remains immature, so will her digestive system. Children with FDS have a digestive system that is dysfunctioning in three primary ways:

1. They produce less stomach acid and digestive enzymes, which chemically help break down and digest food.

2. They have poor muscle tone and fewer muscle contractions of their intestinal and stomach muscles that help mechanically break down food.
3. They have poor circulation in their intestine and stomach lining.

As more and new foods are introduced to the digestive system, more blood is needed to keep the digestive processes moving. When the digestive system is not maturing properly, this isn't happening.

Normally, the stomach is lined with closely linked cells that form a tight barrier against only the smallest of molecules. This protects the stomach against foreign invaders, such as bacteria, viruses, fungi, or parasites. Inadequate blood flow, however, prevents these cells from maintaining a firm seal.

Not only does low blood flow make the stomach more vulnerable to foreign invaders, it allows larger molecules to escape into the bloodstream before they can be broken down to release vitamins and minerals. As a result, nutrients are lost.

This vicious cycle is known as leaky gut syndrome. Kids with a leaky gut can have nutritional deficits even if they eat healthy, nutrient-dense foods all the time. Leaky gut also can cause food sensitivities.

The majority of the immune system's antibodies—about 60 percent—reside in the intestinal wall like soldiers guarding a fortress. They remain peaceable until a foreign invader comes along and threatens to break through and disrupt routine operations. However, these antibodies will jump to the defense if anything comes along that looks suspicious. Large protein molecules from partially digested food that escape from the gut look a lot like menacing bacteria, viruses, and fungi, so the immune system treats them all the same and pummels them with antibodies. When this happens often enough, the body becomes sensitive to these proteins and treats them like enemies. This vicious cycle is how kids with FDS end up sensitive to certain foods.

ACADEMIC SYMPTOMS

Children with FDS are often intelligent—some are exceptionally so—but they still struggle with school. They will get normal or above average grades in some subjects but score below average in others.

BRAIN BALANCE PROFILE: *Gabriel*

A Severe Disconnect Corrects

Gabriel was six when his mother brought him to see me. I was impressed with her right away. She was extremely knowledgeable and had committed all of her time and resources to finding ways to help her son, who was diagnosed with both moderate autism and ADHD.

When I first evaluated Gabriel, he had severe language difficulties. He didn't communicate much and would repetitively say phrases he had heard on the television. It was clear, however, that he had no real understanding of the words he was constantly repeating.

Gabriel would not make eye contact with me. His mother told me that he was this way with everybody. If I turned my back just for a second, he would make a run for it. I was often chasing him down the hall to bring him back to our sessions. He also had no sense of smell and a fast heart rate for his age, which was very puzzling to his pediatrician. He was physically stressed out.

Gabriel unquestionably had the classic signs of autism. I started to work with him by doing a number of physical exercises and sensory stimulation directed at activating his right brain.

Testing also found that Gabriel had moderate to severe sensitivities to a number of foods, most notably dairy, wheat, and eggs. So we took him off these foods and changed his diet in other ways to make it more nutritious.

Six weeks into the program, his mother brought him to a session with tears of joy. "I just had my first real conversation with my son," she said. From that time on, Gabriel showed significant positive changes in his behavior, motor, and academic skills. He also started to get a sense of smell. His mom was thrilled to report, "For the first time I saw him inhale the aroma of freshly baked chocolate chip cookies."

At the end of twelve weeks, his mother brought me his report card. Earlier in the school year he was getting all Rs, for Requires Support. Now he had all Ms, for Meets Expectations. She was ecstatic.

At about this time we also redid blood tests to check his sensitivities. His wheat sensitivity had gone away and he now showed only a slight sensitivity to dairy. This was a sign that his digestive system was functioning better and his immune system was not as hyperactive. His pediatrician reported that his heart rate was now normal.

Many children with ADHD and Asperger's, for example, usually start out with superior verbal skills. They are early word readers. Some children with autism teach themselves how to read at an early age. Some have even astounded their parents by reading words out of a children's book at eighteen months of age!

Other children are exceptional at math operations. They can easily calculate numbers in their head but they have significant difficulty with math reasoning skills.

All these children may start out impressing both parents and teachers with their math and/or reading abilities but as they get to around fourth or fifth grade, they start to have trouble academically. Good readers, for example, will have trouble comprehending what they are reading. Their teachers will find that they cannot understand why the characters in the story are doing or acting a particular way. They have particular difficulty in the pragmatic aspects of language and metaphor. They cannot make inferences. Because of this, they don't derive pleasure from reading and generally avoid reading.

On basic childhood IQ tests, they will show a drastic difference in verbal and nonverbal skills. Typically, children will show a slight difference between these two scores but some children will have a 30-, 40-, or 50-point difference. I have worked with children who have scored 150 in verbal skills—that's genius level—and 70 in nonverbal skills!

How can this be? How can a child have genius-level skills in certain academic areas and mentally retarded levels in others?

The answer to this has eluded and confused educators for years. I lecture to many educators and school psychologists and they admit that this is baffling. This is no surprise, because an understanding of why this happens has never existed before.

We have known for a long time that the growing number of children who have a weakness in comprehension and math reasoning do not create mental images of the words and concepts. Instead of processing the whole or the *gestalt* of the information presented, they tend to connect only to parts of what they read or hear.

The reason this is happening is because comprehension, which is a right brain skill, and word imaging, which is a left brain skill, are not blending. And the reason they are not blending is because the brain is out of sync. The left and right are not communicating.

The symptoms of academic problems that Disconnected Children display are long, but these are some of the more common ones:

Poor oral and written expression
Poor reading and written comprehension
Poor writing skills
Inability to organize
Lack of focus
Reading and spelling problems
Inability to follow directions
Lack of concentration
Difficulty understanding cause and effect
Poor sequencing ability
Confusion when presented with multiple bits of information
Poor social skills

COGNITIVE SYMPTOMS

These are the symptoms that most people associate with learning and behavior disorders and the ones that parents, educators, and health professionals focus on and worry about the most.

They worry about them because they think of ADHD primarily as an attention problem, autism as a communication and socialization problem, and dyslexia as a reading problem.

Only they are not. There is no question that they *are* a problem, but they are not *the* problem. They are only a symptom of the real problem, which is an imbalance between the left and the right hemispheres of the brain.

Cognitive skills are what define a child as an individual with a unique personality. These are the skills that will carve a child's future success in life. They drive how a child will think, learn, rationalize, make decisions, plan, initiate, express emotions, control impulses, establish goals, regulate behavior, and engage in other high-level activities. They are like the brain's boss—the chief executive officer of all functions and operations. This is why cognitive skills are also known as executive functions.

Executive functions are controlled in the prefrontal lobe of the frontal cortex, the slowest to grow and most sophisticated part of the brain.

Acting inappropriately for one's age, an inability to pay attention in school, and issues with social relationships and making friends are signs that this important part of the brain is not developing properly. The symptoms include but are not limited to:

Inappropriate laughing and giggling
Lack of fear, especially in the face of danger
Risk taking
An aversion to being cuddled or held
Sustained unusual or repetitive play
Avoiding eye contact
A preference to play alone
Difficulty in expressing needs
Making wild gestures
Insistence on everything being the same
Difficulty interacting with others
Difficulty setting goals and prioritizing
Difficulty controlling emotions
Difficulty learning, remembering, and paying attention
Poor motor control
Inability to monitor own actions

You will notice that a number of these symptoms have appeared in other parts of this chapter. This is just another example of the interrelationship of what is going on in the brains of Disconnected Children.

Lack of synchronization, or what doctors call temporal coherence, between the two hemispheres of the brain and/or various large areas of the central nervous system, leads to a disconnect in functions. It's like various lightbulbs burning out in a big room filled with lamps.

When the two hemispheres cannot bind and share information, it forces a reliance on one side of the brain. This is why the abilities that reside in the strong functioning side of the brain can appear exaggerated. This does not mean that the brain is damaged. It's just too slow in one half and too fast in the other. This can be fixed. The room can get brighter again.

In order to make the fix permanent, however, the underlying cause or causes of the problem need to be addressed. This is controversial territory and it is coming up next.

❀ BRAIN BALANCE PROFILE: *Robbie and Paul*

AMAZING PROGRESS IN JUST SIX MONTHS

Robbie was age three and his brother, Paul, was just sixteen months old when his parents came to see me after both boys were diagnosed with severe autism.

Their mother, Regina, an exercise physiologist and physical therapist, took all precautions from the moment she planned her pregnancies, and her deliveries were normal. She never had her children vaccinated, and she fed the family only organic food. Nevertheless, Regina and her husband noticed something wasn't quite right with their children almost from the start.

Both boys were delayed in developmental milestones. Robbie started to crawl and walk late. When we met, he was completely nonverbal. Paul could not crawl or walk and could only scoot on his bottom.

Paul's symptoms were the more severe. He would scream for dear life when anyone other than a parent approached him, and he would thrust himself out of his mother's arms when he was unhappy. He would sit and smash his head against the floor, and his lack of reaction to pain was alarming to his parents. Robbie could follow basic instructions but he lacked expression and appeared unaware of what was going on around him. He had a reduced sensitivity to sound and touch. These and other symptoms indicated both boys had a right brain delay. Urine and blood tests confirmed a number of food sensitivities as well as vitamin, amino acid, and mineral deficiencies.

We tailored an exercise and sensory stimulation program for both boys specific to their individual right brain imbalance. We also addressed their dietary problems with an elimination diet and supplement program. Paul, though more severely autistic, responded more quickly because he was the youngest. In just six months, Paul was standing on a trampoline, laughing, reciting the alphabet, and recognizing himself in the mirror for the first time. By that same time, Robbie was talking and expressing himself, though it took him longer to catch up to where he should have been for his age. Both boys were well on their way to realizing a normal childhood.

4

WHAT'S CAUSING IT ALL?

Let's Stop Confusing the Issue

■

If young bodies are in bad shape, what
about the brains that are attached to them?

—JANE HEALEY, PHD

■

W ALK AROUND ANY neighborhood in the late afternoon and
chances are you'll see a lot of things—trees, cars, houses, sidewalks.
What you won't see, however, are many kids outside playing.

When I was a kid, children were always playing outdoors. You'd see
them on their bikes, on roller skates, shooting baskets, playing street
hockey, and even climbing trees.

Not these days. It's not that there are fewer children. In many neigh-
borhoods there actually are more. Where you'll find them, though, is
inside watching television, playing computer games, or lazing in a chair
text messaging their friends.

This is about the worst thing they could be doing for their growing
brains.

The questions that I always get when I'm talking to parents and educators are, *Why? Why are so many children getting autism and ADHD? Why
are classrooms filled with kids on medication? Why did this happen to my child?*

Answering these questions isn't always that easy, not because I don't
have an explanation—I do—but because so many people are confused and

misinformed about the nature of neurological childhood disorders. This is quite unfortunate because it only adds to the anxiety and despair of those trying to deal with these conditions at home and at school. And this is why this chapter is so important. You can use my home-based Brain Balance Program and get results but you're not going to be able to make those results permanent unless you understand the underlying causes and do the best in your power to correct them.

After fifteen years of research and working with mentally dysfunctional children, I can say without hesitation that the underlying causes of the vast majority of the problems we are seeing today can be found in the environment.

Before I get to what they are, however, I want to address a few things that are confusing the issue.

WHAT OTHERS ARE SAYING

Many so-called experts would like you to believe that the increase in these problems is being overdramatized. They say it only seems that the incidence of autism and ADHD is climbing because better and earlier diagnoses make it appear that way. There may be a little truth to this, but it is not a plausible explanation.

There are others who propose that these problems are purely genetically based. Again this is not plausible because any scientist will attest that genetic problems don't explode onto the scene like this. The rise has just been too fast and too specific.

One reason for this assumption is the likelihood of autism in identical twins. Statistics show that if one twin gets autism, the chance that the other will get it is between 60 and 80 percent. Again, this doesn't make sense. Identical twins have identical genes. So, if autism were genetic, then the chance of both twins getting it would have to be closer to 100 percent.

Besides, if genetics were the cause, the incidence of autism would be going down, not up, because autistic adults generally don't marry, and when they do, they generally don't have children.

Another genetically linked contention has to do with the numerous studies showing that more than 50 percent of children diagnosed with ADHD and all other neurobehavioral disorders also meet the medically established diagnostic criteria for one or more other psychiatric dysfunction such as mood, anxiety, learning, or behavior disorders. In this case, experts theorize that these disorders have similar underlying genetic mutations, although there is no evidence to support such a contention. Again, this is not plausible. It is unlikely that one small child could possibly have two or three different psychiatric conditions simultaneously. Besides, I've already shown that all of these disorders are really one and the same.

The genetic explanation—or to be blunt, excuse—is not only misrepresented, it is a disservice to parents because it is another way of saying that there is no hope for a cure.

This is not to say that genes don't play a role in the development of these conditions. In fact, there is evidence of a genetic tendency. The tendency, however, is epigenetic, meaning that there exists environmental influences so powerful that they can turn on, turn off, or even alter a gene's expression. Simply put, negative influences in the environment can make genes more vulnerable.

I believe—and there is plenty of supporting evidence to prove—that the epidemic rise in neurobehavioral and neuroacademic disorders is being caused by negative influences in the environment—namely, many of the practices that make up the typical modern American lifestyle.

This isn't hard to see when viewed in the context of the social changes that have occurred primarily in the United States during the last ten to twenty years. I see the major contributors as:

Lack of physical exercise
Overweight and obesity
Absentee parenting
Television and computer games
Stressful pregnancies and births
Stressful lifestyles
Environmental toxins
Inadequate nutrition

Each of these negative influences is interfering with the positive environmental stimulation the brain needs to grow and strengthen. The most egregious is physical inactivity.

BODY AND BRAIN ARE CODEPENDENT

At one time scientists believed that there was no relationship between the developing brain and the developing body. We now know this is not the case. Body and mind are codependent. In fact, there is a whole new scientific concept gaining popularity in the artificial intelligence and robotics community known as embodiment, which states that the development of intelligence without a body may, in fact, be impossible. The brain is dependent on the body to provide the stimulation necessary for growth as much as the body is dependent on the brain to send out the neurotransmitters that signal the muscles to move. As I explained in Chapter 2, the brain's only continuous source of stimulation comes from the body's resistance to gravity and this happens through movement. Without movement as its primary source of stimulation, the brain will struggle to grow.

Philip Teitelbaum, PhD, an expert on human movement patterns at the University of Florida at Gainesville, recognized the interdependence of body and brain when he studied the physical development of children who were later diagnosed with autism. As infants and toddlers, he found, autistic children use unusual strategies for locomotion. They do not roll over, sit up, crawl, or learn to walk like normal children. He explained that it is as if the parts of the brain that control movement are not properly connected.

"We tend to think that [autism] is a problem with the mind," Dr. Teitelbaum said in an interview with the *New York Times*. "Now that we are really beginning to see how the brain works, we know that the mind is embodied. Body is part of the mind and there's no way to separate it."

Just as the muscles of the body develop with exercise, the cells in the brain develop with exercise. The brain is activity dependent, so the more activity it gets, the more it will grow in size and density. The quality and quantity of movement of all the muscles are directly correlated to the quality and quantity of functional capacity in the brain.

What this all means is that if children don't move their muscles, their brains are not going to grow. There is no question that the way children use and move their bodies, both consciously and unconsciously, has a profound effect on the brain.

SEDENTARY CHILDREN

Today's young people are the most out of shape and overweight in all of history. As a group, they are so unfit that in 1989 the U.S. Army had to relax its physical requirements in basic training. An official at the time stated, "Young people coming into the military now have spent more time in front of the TV than on the tennis court or softball field." And that was twenty years ago!

Since then it has gotten even worse as evidenced by the other epidemic that is threatening the health of America's children: obesity. American children as a whole not only are the most physically unfit in the world but are also the fattest.

The obesity rate of children between the ages of two to five has doubled in the last thirty years and it has tripled in kids ages six through eleven. More than 17 percent of our children—that's more than 9 million kids—are considered overweight.

Scientists have been watching kids get fatter and exercise less since the 1980s. They can show a direct correlation between an increase in the percentage of body fat and a decrease in physical exercise, especially during the last decade. Not coincidentally, during the past decade, we have also seen the sharpest increase in the percentage of children with severe behavioral problems, poor socialization skills, learning disabilities, attention problems, and children on Ritalin and other powerful psychiatric drugs. During the same time, teachers report, children's attention spans have gotten shorter, classroom behavior has gotten worse, and children are much slower at processing information.

Obesity is just as dangerous to the developing brain as inactivity. For starters, obesity and inactivity are both associated with decreased muscle mass and muscle tone, especially in the big muscles (postural anti-gravity muscles) that create proper posture and a good gait. Decreased muscle tone, in turn, is directly related to decreased stimulation to the brain, especially to the centers of higher learning and thinking.

Also, researchers in Toronto found that the brains of children who eat a high-fat diet are not getting enough glucose—that is, brain food. As a result, the kids in this study showed impaired memory and poor concentration. It is, they explained, as if fat is blocking the glucose pathway to the brain and starving it. The researchers expressed concern that this could permanently damage developing neural pathways.

The saddest thing about all this is that these troubles are not necessarily the fault of the kids themselves. It is really a familial issue.

WHO'S RAISING OUR CHILDREN?

What I am about to say will cause some controversy, but I am going to say it nevertheless. I believe, and there is evidence to back me up, that the parents' own health and lifestyle unknowingly and unintentionally are actually at the root of the problem.

Most children who end up with some type of neurological dysfunction start out life (and brain development) in the care of someone other than a parent because both mother and father are working. Parenting often becomes a second job, or what I call "moonlighting" parenting.

Because of the need or desire to maintain two careers, today's parents do not spend time with their children as families did in the past. Owing to time restraints, parents do not talk to their kids as much as they did ten years ago, or read to them, or spend time just being together.

The all-important mother-child bond is shared with an outside third party. Recent statistics show that more than half of America's one-year-olds are spending their days with someone other than their mothers. Three-quarters of school-age children and two-thirds of preschoolers have mothers in the labor force. This indicates that a large percentage of schoolchildren come home after school to a house without a parent or guardian.

Other statistics show that 50 percent of two-wage-earning parents or single mothers do not have adequate day care available to them. Additionally, English is frequently a second language for many day care workers, meaning these children are learning to speak English from a non-English-speaking adult. I have noticed in situations like this that some children are learning to speak with slight foreign accents.

Teachers say they can see the effects in the classroom. When parents are not around, the television, computer, and video games become the surrogate babysitter. Sedentary activities breed sedentary activities.

Many parents of children with learning and behavior problems are overweight and out of shape, and this has a major influence on their child's weight and physical activity. This strongly suggests that many parents are unaware of good, basic nutritional concepts and they are not feeding their children, or themselves, properly.

It is a widely accepted fact that children learn to use and move their bodies by subconsciously modeling their parents' movements. It is not unusual at all to see children who walk and talk exactly like their parents. This has nothing to do with genetics. It's imitation.

Therefore, if the parents do not use their bodies enough or properly, which, by the way, will decrease their own brainpower, then their children won't either. They will just repeat what they know from their parents. With adult physical fitness at an all-time low and obesity above an unprecedented 60 percent of the adult population, it is easy to assume that there are a lot of parents who are not setting a great example.

TV DULLS THE BRAIN

Too much TV is bad for both the brain and the body. Studies show that when kids sit around watching television, activity in the brain slows. Watching TV for hours on end actually promotes atrophy of muscles, primarily the muscles near the spine (postural antigravity muscles) that promote proper posture and a good gait. Atrophy decreases muscle tone, which decreases the amount of stimulation to the brain, especially to the frontal lobes, the center of higher learning and thinking.

There has been so much research on the negatives of watching too much TV that the American Academy of Pediatrics nearly ten years ago recommended that youngsters under the age of two should not watch any television at all. More recent research has found that every hour preschoolers spend in front of the TV boosts their risk of developing ADHD later in life by 10 percent.

Another study found that children who watched television for four or more hours a day have a higher ratio of body fat than children who watch one to three hours of TV. Conversely, children who watch television for an hour or less a day had the lowest ratio of body fat.

Now consider this finding when wondering what is happening to the brains of today's young people: The average high school graduate will have spent 15,000 to 18,000 hours watching television but only 12,000 hours in school.

▶ *TV and Aggressive Behavior*

There are many professionals and parents who dismiss reports that violent TV can result in violent behavior, but recent neuroscientific research has finally proven how it can happen. Researchers at Columbia University Medical Center studied brain activity in a group of children as they watched movies depicting violence and found that the part of the brain that suppresses violent behavior became less active. This could render children less able to control aggressive behavior.

In the same study, the researchers also found that viewing violence made areas of the brain that plan behavior less active. This finding further suggests that exposure to violence can diminish the brain's ability to control behavior. Neither of these changes in brain activity, however, occurred when the children watched nonviolent but equally engaging video games or movies depicting horror scenes or physical activity.

Another study at the Indiana University School of Medicine evaluated the brains of seventy-one students after watching violence and found that it reduced activity in the right frontal lobe, the area that controls behavior and higher learning skills, among others. They also found that activity was slower in students with symptoms associated with ADHD.

COMPUTER GAMES AND THE BRAIN

Many parents believe that playing computer games helps kids improve their minds but this isn't necessarily so. Although research shows that playing on a computer does help some cognitive skills, it appears that the negative effects far outweigh the positives.

For example, video games don't teach children in the same way as traditional classroom learning or learning through life experiences. One researcher illustrated that the only valuable skill it gives children is the ability to recognize icons and symbols.

Researchers have also found that teenagers who play violent video games experience real-life physical symptoms. Their heart rate and respiration get faster and body temperature goes up. These games, as well as violent movies, can also affect the parts of the brain that control aggressive behavior.

One study has found that playing computer games may stunt brain development. Researchers in Japan used a highly specialized mind-mapping technology to monitor brain activities in hundreds of teenagers playing Nintendo and compared the results to the brain scans of hundreds of kids doing simple arithmetic calculations. The researchers found that the only brain activity going on in the brains of the teens playing on the computer was in the areas that control vision and movement. They found no activity in the frontal lobes.

By contrast, the researchers observed that both the left and the right hemispheres of the kids' brains doing the arithmetic were highly active.

At the very least, this indicates that parents should monitor the time children spend playing on the computer. Surveys show, however, that most parents don't monitor their children's computer time. Even parents who monitor TV time don't necessarily monitor computer time.

POOR NUTRITION

Considering how much emphasis there is on food and the expanding American waistline, our dietary problems are only escalating. The problem isn't just what we are eating and feeding our children; it has a lot to do with what is and isn't in the food itself. The composition of the foods we typically eat—even fruits and vegetables—has changed tremendously, and mostly for the worse.

Farmed foods no longer provide the abundant nutrient levels that they supplied in the past. The rapid turnover of crops and overutilization of farmland continue to deplete minerals in the soil. According to one report, an average of 250 million tons of pesticides are used worldwide each year on crops that supply the fruits, vegetables, and grains we eat and feed to our children. This does not include the millions of tons of herbicides and fungicides used in the agricultural system.

Nonorganic food farms—which are, by far, the majority—feed hormones, antibiotics, and suboptimal feed to the cattle and livestock that end up as our protein.

Soil, water, and air pollution continue to be a major problem that affects everyone, but the toxic effects they have on Disconnected Children can be quite profound.

In the last twenty-five to thirty years, food has become more and more processed with tremendous increases in sugar, refined carbohydrates, and the worst kinds of fats. Family dinners often consist of prepackaged meals too high in fat, artificial additives, and preservatives. And of course, there is the tremendous increase in the consumption of unhealthy soft drinks.

Fast-food restaurants are a common substitute for a real meal, offering only further nutritional depletion. These kinds of meals offer the lowest quality, highest processing, and the two most common "vegetables" in too many kids' diets—French fries and ketchup! Plus, fast food is loaded with salt and saturated fat.

Most parents don't recognize the detrimental effects a poor diet has on the developing brain, especially in children who already have Functional Disconnection Syndrome. It can impact everything that is already troublesome for a child with FDS—behavior, cognitive or academic achievement, sensory processing, gross and fine motor skills, equilibrium, a wacky immune system, and normal everyday body functions, such as digestion and elimination.

MOTHER-CHILD STRESS

It's well known that the mother provides the environment that helps her baby develop in the womb, so it goes without saying that the mom-to-be's lifestyle has a profound effect on fetal brain development. What is less known is that the mom-to-be's lifestyle can have a similar impact on her child's brain development after birth. If a baby's brain is developing too slowly in the womb, it means an infant will begin life having to play "catch up," which will show up later as delays in development.

Research indicates that a pregnant woman's current and previous levels of physical and mental health, physical activity, eating habits, sleeping patterns, hormonal balance, and stress level can later affect her child's behavior and intellectual capacity. Also, anything that negatively affects a pregnant woman's hormone levels and autonomic, immune, and nervous system functions can negatively impact the brain of a developing fetus. These include toxins, bad nutrition, alcohol, recreational drugs, medications taken during pregnancy, smoking, and stress.

Even things a mother can't control can be potentially damaging to her child's brain. One study of 188 mothers of autistic children found a common link: They all experienced a major life stress, such as the death of someone close or job loss, during their last trimester.

When and how behavioral traits originate in the womb is the subject of ongoing research. For example, several studies on temperament measured heart rate and movement of an infant while in the womb and at birth. Results showed that very active fetuses tend to become irritable infants. Those with irregular sleep/wake patterns in the womb sleep more poorly as young infants. Also fetuses with high heart rates become unpredictable inactive babies. It appears that this is the result of increased levels of stress hormones during pregnancy.

Researchers are even seeing a link between the incidence of ADHD and women who have their first child after the age of thirty-five. In one study, for instance, researchers reviewed the medical histories of 300 hyperactive children and 300 normal children. They found that, during pregnancy, the mothers of children with ADHD were older, generally in poorer health, had higher levels of toxins in the blood, were delivering a first child, and went through longer labor (more than thirteen hours) than mothers of the normal children. They were also more likely to have had high blood pressure during pregnancy.

TRAUMATIC BIRTH

Traveling through the birth canal may be the most dangerous journey a human will ever take. Modern medicine has not been able to make the journey much safer. In fact, approximately 10 percent of all stillborn births in the United States are the result of neurological damage to the brain stem caused by the medically assisted delivery process.

Unfortunately, more frequently there are subtle injuries occurring at birth that go unrecognized by physicians who are unfamiliar with how to diagnose and/or treat these types of birth-related injuries. Usually, these injuries are to the cervical spine. If left untreated, they can result in significant developmental and functional neurological problems that can persist through life.

These injuries often result in decreased motion of cervical vertebrate and cervical muscles, which provide the largest amount of stimulation to the brain and body. Robbing the brain of this stimulation can cause significant imbalances in brain activity, which will show up later as below-average IQ, specific learning disabilities, behavioral problems, immune challenges, sensory deficits, or poor muscular abilities.

When the high percentage of children who probably suffer from this type of trauma is considered, it may actually be one of the largest causes of higher cognitive and behavioral problems in children.

■ Why More Boys Have Problems ■

FOUR out of five children diagnosed with autism are males. There is also a much higher incidence of boys with ADHD than girls. Evidence indicates this has to do with several factors:

Boys are most susceptible to environmental toxins during prenatal development and during the first two years of life. This is when the right brain is developing. Boys have a larger right brain than left brain and are generally more dependent on right hemisphere abilities than girls. Because the right brain develops first, lack of physical movement and exercise in the toddler years will have a more negative impact on boys than girls. Boys are more affected by maternal prenatal stress than girls. This affects the development of strong male characteristics, which means the right side of the brain may not grow as large as it normally would.

Girls have a larger bridge that connects the left and the right hemispheres. This helps compensate in the presence of negative environmental factors. ■

INJURY AND ILLNESS

A common injury that can interfere with brain development in children, especially infants, is a neck injury. Babies and children have extremely large heads for their body size and they sit on very small necks. The muscles of the neck are very immature and weak and cannot support an infant's head. This makes it extremely easy for a child to suffer a whiplash injury to the cervical spine. Unfortunately, this type of injury goes unnoticed because infants can't speak and most pediatricians generally are not adept at examining their necks for subtle trauma.

Whiplash can occur from an adult picking a child up improperly, pulling a child, hitting a child, or from the child striking his head in a fall. If a child strikes his head, face, or mouth hard enough to cause a cut or bruise, it most likely will cause some degree of whiplash. This may result in subtle or severe muscle spasms.

Since pediatricians are not on the lookout for this type of injury, a parent needs to speak up and ask the doctor to examine the neck during regular visits. If a child falls or if a parent has even the smallest suspicion that there could be a neck injury, the child should be seen by a health professional trained in such injuries. This would be a chiropractor or an osteopathic physician.

Any injury that causes a child to go through a long period of sedentary convalescence or limits the use of the large muscles can also cause developmental delay. Once started, such a delay may continually leave the child behind and may cause difficulties in school and/or immature behavior that may be seen as a behavioral or emotional problem. If there is not an effort to specifically intervene to normalize the nervous system delay, the child may never "catch up" and the problem could persist into adulthood.

Another common injury in infants can result from incorrect placement in a car seat. Safety checks have found that up to 85 percent of caregivers use car safety seats improperly. In this case, even a minor motor vehicle accident can result in severe injury to the child.

Although musculoskeletal injuries and their potential neurological consequences may be by far the greatest risk, childhood illness is also a potential problem.

Any illness that causes prolonged inactivity can result in developmental delays.

Chronic ear infections can dampen sound transmission, which can alter sensory input. An eye injury can do the same to the visual processing centers. Children with chronic ear infections are often prescribed many different powerful antibiotics. The American Medical Association and other top medical physicians express concern that young children are given too many antibiotics. When antibiotics are given unnecessarily or incorrectly, stronger bacteria can develop in later illnesses and make them harder to fight.

. . .

BRAIN BALANCE PROFILE: *Allan*

LIKE LIFE IS BEGINNING ANEW

Allan was a child who came into the world screaming and never seemed to stop. Though a happy and "busy" baby, his parents watched him turn into an angry and disagreeable toddler. Sensing he was not a typical child, they took him to a psychologist, who diagnosed ADHD. He was three.

This marked a long journey of expensive evaluations, special education, social skills classes, inclusion therapy, and neurofeedback, just to name a few, that exhausted his parents and took a toll on life for the whole family. His disheartened parents watched him only get worse.

When we first met, Allan was a wildly erratic eight-year-old, as many children with this diagnosis are. He was so disruptive at home and school that he required constant supervision. He couldn't even ride the bus with the other kids.

Brain Balance brought the first big breakthrough in Allan's behavior. After twelve weeks, he was riding the regular school bus with his siblings and no longer required an aide to assist him after special ed. His marks went up in all his subjects. By the time summer rolled around, Allan was in summer camp for the first time in his life and was making new friends.

Brain Balance showed the first significant change in Allan's behavior, according to his parents. "Our family and friends marvel at the delightful 'new' Allan," they said. "We thank you, and although Allan is too young to appreciate what has happened to him, someday he will thank you as well."

5

LEFT BRAIN, RIGHT BRAIN

One Can't Grow Strong Without the Other

■

Most parents are told that their children will not improve and they lose all
hope. I tell parents to look at my boys. I say, 'If they can get better so can yours.'

—REGINA, MOTHER OF TWO BOYS DIAGNOSED WITH SEVERE AUTISM

■

Fｒｏｍ ｔｈｅ ｍｏｍｅｎｔ the brain starts growing in the womb, to the
moment of birth, and up to about age two, brain development is concentrated on the right side. This is a vulnerable period of time for the
brain, as it is particularly susceptible to some of the negative environmental influences that you read about in Chapter 4. Anything that interferes with prenatal development, the birthing process, or healthy growth
during the first two years of life can affect how the right brain grows. This
is probably the major reason why a right brain deficiency is more common than a left brain deficiency.

HOW THE RIGHT BRAIN WORKS

The right brain holds the big picture view of the world. It is great at seeing the whole, but not the parts. It sees the forest, so to speak, but can't
see the trees.

The right brain is also in charge of moving the big muscles. It controls posture and gait. It is also the spatial side of the brain. It allows a child to feel himself in space. It controls balance and what is known as proprioception, the ability to know where the body is in relationship to gravity and in relationship to self and others.

The right hemisphere is the brain's nonverbal communicator. It reads and interprets body posture, facial expression, tone of voice, and understands what a person is thinking or feeling. Nonverbal communication is the foundation of socialization, so the right brain is the social brain. Because the right brain is nonverbal, it learns subconsciously or subliminally. A child doesn't always realize he is learning—after all, everything is a new learning experience to an infant and toddler—but this does not make it less important.

Nonverbal ability is also the foundation of verbal communication that will develop later on the left side of the brain.

The right side of the brain is the more emotional side. It helps a child feel his own emotions and also read emotions in others. This is what we call emotional intelligence, or EQ.

The right brain also operates the sensory controls, so it senses and feels the whole body. This is because the right side borders the part of the brain known as the insula cortex, in which a child feels the internal sensations from the gut, heart, and lungs that allow him to feel emotion.

The right brain is also the empathetic brain. Once a child can read emotions in himself, he will start to develop the ability to read the same emotions in other people through nonverbal communication.

The right brain is also very attuned to the sense of smell and taste. It is responsible for determining if a smell is good, and therefore the person or object is good, or the smell is bad, and therefore the person or object should be avoided. It is also responsible for receiving information from the auditory system.

The right brain is governed by what is known as avoidance behavior, so it is the cautious brain. It is the part of the brain that keeps a child safe. Before the curious left brain can approach something, the right brain has to give its consent that it is safe. Being in charge of avoidance makes the right brain the keeper of negative emotions, such as fear, anger, and disgust.

Because the right side of the brain is cautious and sensory, it is responsible for attention. It controls impulses. It will stop a child from doing something, especially when it is socially inappropriate.

The right brain likes new or novel situations or locations. It hates to do the same thing over and over. Routine bores it easily.

The right hemisphere helps to control the immune system. It inhibits it and prevents it from overreacting, so it doesn't turn on its own protective antibodies.

The right hemisphere also controls most life-supporting automatic reactions, especially digestion. It controls the pacemaker in the heart that regulates heartbeat.

■ Savant Syndrome ■

SAVANTS are children, usually boys, who despite serious mental and sometimes even physical disabilities, display a remarkable talent. In some cases, this talent is considered genius. Most often it occurs in children diagnosed with autism, a right brain deficiency.

Savant syndrome is the result of a greatly magnified or enhanced left brain skill that is also mirrored with deeply weak right brain abilities. In fact, some savants can have a genius-level skill but otherwise cannot communicate. Some are even considered to be retarded.

One of the more common skills of a savant is a remarkable ability to play music, even though the child cannot read music and never took a lesson. Some savants have been known to draw incredibly accurate reproductions of objects or locations from memory. They include remarkable detail, showing exceptional fine motor skill.

The musical ability comes from enhanced left brain ability that results in perfect pitch, the unique talent to perfectly reproduce a note when heard. It is rare in the general population, even among highly skilled musicians. Mozart was actually believed to be an autistic savant. Mozart's music is believed to be unique because it contains an unusually high number of high-frequency notes, much higher than any other music. High-frequency sounds stimulate the left brain.

Other typical savant skills are a remarkable ability to calculate numbers, and an amazing memory for dates or details, such as baseball statistics.

Probably the most well-known savant today is Kim Peek, the inspiration for Barry Morrow's 1988 hit movie *Rain Man*. Peek, who was born in 1951, can read at an amazing speed and has total recall of almost all the details in every book he has read, even though he scores below average on a general IQ test. He reportedly has read more than 12,000 books.

Peek is not considered autistic. He was born with an abnormal cerebellum, the result of a lack of the bridge that connects the two hemispheres
of the brain—a true structural disconnection syndrome.

▶ When the Right Goes Wrong

Children with right hemisphere deficits don't feel their bodies well.
They have poor muscle tone, especially of the large postural muscles
near the spine. The most glaring symptom is an odd gait.

They will also have delayed and poor gross motor skills, including poor
balance, rhythm, and coordination. This means they will trip and fall a lot
for no good reason.

This oddness can also be noted in their social skills. They may say inappropriate things without understanding why they are wrong. They often
have a hard time making friends.

These kids are usually very picky eaters. They avoid foods because they
don't have a normal sense of smell or taste. They don't eat foods that kids
normally like, especially sweets.

The right brain is about reading people and situations but the left brain
is about reading words. So, when children do not develop the right brain's
nonverbal skills, it makes learning verbal skills difficult or even impossible. Children with right brain deficiencies may be good at reading words
but will not be good at interpreting what they are reading. They may also
be good with numbers but be bad at higher-level math skills.

Children with right hemisphere weaknesses have poor attention. They
are impulsive and anxious. They also tend to be compulsive.

Autoimmune disorders, such as allergies and asthma, often go hand in
hand with a right brain imbalance. These children are often very sensitive
to the environment, certain foods, and may have a number of contact allergies. When the right side cannot suppress the immune system, it can
cause inflammation in the body and brain. This can become chronic.
These children will have poor digestion. A rapid heartbeat is also common.

Right brain deficiencies are often diagnosed as:

ADD
ADHD
Asperger's syndrome
Autism

Tourette syndrome
Obsessive compulsive disorder (OCD)
Oppositional defiant disorder (ODD)
Nonverbal learning disorder (NLD)
Pervasive developmental disorder (PDD)
Developmental coordination disorder (DCD)
Conduct disorder (CD)

■ The Analytical Brain Versus the Creative Brain ■

CONVENTIONAL wisdom says that artists and writers are right-brained because they are creative, and computer wizards and accountants are left-brained because they are analytical. However, this is not entirely correct.

Many of the world's great musicians and artists, for example, are considered to be highly left-brained. There is a logical explanation for this.

Playing music and doing fine art most often are about following a pattern that has already been created. For example, in the case of learning to play an instrument, it is following a musical score; in the case of art, it is copying something from nature. In fact, many great artists who do still-life paintings or portraits have to have the subject in front of them; they would have great difficulty painting a scene from memory.

Abstract art, however, is different. It is truly unique because it is not based on reality. This makes abstract art a right brain ability. This is where the concept of creativity and the right brain originated. Thinking or painting or creating something completely new, unique, or novel is what the right brain does.

So rest assured. Your child can be either left-brained or right-brained and still be creative. ■

HOW THE LEFT BRAIN WORKS

The left hemisphere sees the world in small pictures, like the stills that make up a movie. It ignores the whole and zeroes in on the details. It breaks things into small pieces and examines them.

The left brain controls the small muscles or fine motor skills. Everything done with the hands and fingers, feet and toes, such as tying shoes or playing the piano, are left brain skills. The left brain moves the small muscles of the throat and mouth in rapid sequence so a child can speak. Likewise, it translates the rapidly differing sounds of letters and syllables into language. The left hemisphere is the verbal side of the brain. Everything that has to do with language resides here. Reading, writing, speaking, and interpretation all take place here. It reads individual words in a sentence and translates their meaning, letter by letter, and syllable by syllable. The left brain is the literal brain, understanding only one primary meaning of a word.

Because it is attuned to words, the left is the conscious side of the brain. It is involved in every conscious move the body makes. It is also involved in conscious thoughts—a child talks to herself with the left brain. When your child is doing her homework—reading a book, doing a math problem, or memorizing a poem—she is using her left brain. The left is the linear and logical brain. It works out basic math operations, arithmetic, calculating, and remembering numbers in a sequence.

The left brain is good at pattern recognition skills—that is, figuring out what comes next in a sequence, or figuring out a pattern. Language develops because of pattern recognition skills. This is believed to be the reason why children can learn a new language so easily. Learning to play a musical instrument is a pattern skill. It also involves using fine motor skills, which are controlled on the left. Computer games and video games are all about pattern recognition skills. The left brain loves computer games.

The left brain is about systemizing; it's linear and logical in its thinking. It likes to examine things one at a time and in order. It likes basic science and math and other logical pursuits.

It is the thinking brain. It loves to do the same routine over and over. It hates new things.

The left brain is very curious. It is responsible for intelligence, especially verbal intelligence, and is more measured by traditional IQ tests than the right brain.

Behaviorally, the left brain controls what we call approach behavior. It wants to approach a situation to study all the details and figure out a pattern and remember that pattern. Emotionally, it is in charge of positive emotions, and motivation—happiness, having fun, get-up-and-go.

The left brain is specialized to hear high-frequency sounds, which change rapidly, and visually process highly detailed input, which takes longer, so its timing must be perfect in order to compensate for these different speed requirements.

Like the right brain, the left brain also helps control the immune system. It activates it to fight off infections and toxins. It stimulates the growth and development of immune tissue called lymphoid tissue that houses white blood cells and other immune-mediated chemicals. It activates the immune system to produce antibodies to fight off foreign invaders. When a child is sick and has an infection, the left hemisphere mobilizes the immune system to fight it off. It also helps regulate some of the body's automatic functions, such as heart rhythm.

▶ When the Left Gets Out of Rhythm

The signs of a left brain deficiency are usually more subtle than a right brain problem and can often go undetected until a child is in school.

These children may appear kind of shy and even withdrawn and may not be as motivated to want to do the things that typical kids like to do. They often prefer to hang out around the house than go out to play with friends. Some may be kind of sullen and sad. In fact, depression is believed to be a result of decreased activity in the left side of the brain.

These are the kids who were usually slow to start speaking. They may not be good verbally and may not like to talk a lot. Or they may mess up their sentences when speaking, making it hard to understand them.

Poor language skills are a hallmark of a left brain imbalance, especially as a child gets older. These children have problems with reading and spelling because they can't identify the sounds of letters. This can show up in their speaking ability as well. All this can be the result of a problem with processing words and sound. Not only does this affect reading and speaking skills, but these children can be bad at music and may not be able to carry a tune. They may have problems with many subjects, especially basic math, because they are poor with details. This includes fine detailing they do with their hands. This becomes most obvious as very bad handwriting.

Children with left brain imbalances are often very concerned with how they look and dress. They may have unique abilities to read people and situations. They can be very social if they get over their shyness and insecurities. They may be very good athletes, and people and teachers usually like them a lot. They tend to be popular and leaders outside the classroom.

Children with left brain imbalances are prone to chronic infections, like colds and ear infections. They may also have an abnormal or irregular heartbeat, called an arrhythmia.

Left brain deficiencies are often diagnosed as:

Dyslexia
Processing disorders
Central auditory processing disorder
Dyspraxia
Dysgraphia (poor handwriting)
Learning disability
Language disorder
Reading disorder
Acalculia (poor calculating skill)
Selective mutism

■ Left Versus Right ■

HERE is an easy way to remember the activities that reside in each side of the brain. Think of the body as a car and the brain as the engine. The left brain is like the gas pedal, and the right brain is like the brake.

LEFT BRAIN	RIGHT BRAIN
Small picture	Big picture
Verbal communication	Nonverbal communication
Small muscle control	Large muscle control
IQ	EQ
Word reading	Comprehension
Math calculations	Math reasoning
Processing information	Interpreting information
Conscious actions	Unconscious actions
Positive emotions	Negative emotions
High-frequency sound	Low-frequency sound
Low-frequency light	High-frequency light
Receiving auditory input	Interpreting auditory input
Linear and logical thinking	Understanding abstract concepts
Curious and impulsive actions	Cautious and safe actions

Likes routine, sameness	Likes newness, novelty
Activates immunity	Suppresses immunity
	Spatial awareness
	Senses of taste and smell
	Social skills
	Digestion

BRAIN BALANCE PROFILE: *Lori*

HER SEVERE PROBLEMS ARE OVER

For Lori, life had not been good from day one.

She had a severe traumatic birth caused by cord strangulation and placenta tearing prior to delivery. As an infant, she developed much too slowly and was irritated by severe eczema from head to toe. She was delayed in all her milestones, including extremely poor muscle development. At age five, she was diagnosed with profound autism.

When we met Lori at age seven, she was so developmentally challenged that her parents feared they'd have to institutionalize her. She had no sense of danger and her parents were in constant fear that she'd bolt out the door and into traffic.

She suffered from migraines and had a constant twitch on her left side. She was severely underweight, aggressive, and could say only a few words. Because of her hyperactivity, she could not sleep through the night. She had almost stopped interacting with others altogether. She had had so many urinary tract infections that she became allergic to antibiotics. On top of it all, she was diagnosed with a rare heart valve problem at age six.

After three weeks on Brain Balance, her mother came in thrilled— Lori had slept through the night for the first time in five years! But that was just the beginning of her progress. After six months on Brain Balance, her twitching ceased, she was speaking more and more each day, she was making eye contact for the first time in her life, and her parents no longer had to worry about her bolting into traffic. Her muscle and coordination improved to such a degree that she was now even riding her bike.

The best news came from her developmental pediatrician, who

tested her and found that she had jumped from the mental growth of a two-year-old to that of a six-year-old.

These days, her parents report, Lori is much the normal little girl. "She is full of life and involved in life," her mom told us. There is no more aggression, she is growing and gaining weight, she's joined the Girl Scouts, and she's singing in the church choir. She loves to go camping and hiking and enjoys going to school.

"I can drop her off with other people and not have to mention her history or medical background for fear of her melting down," says her mom. "The migraines are gone and there are no more constant infections. She is affectionate, loving, and she smiles a lot."

So do her parents.

THE MELILLO
AT-HOME
BRAIN BALANCE
PROGRAM

6

RECONNECTING THE BRAIN

The Ten Principles of the Brain Balance Program

■

Tears of joy come when I think about the progress
Brenda has made. She speaks. She moves more fluidly.
She expresses her needs. She is a new little person.

—CARLA P., BRENDA'S MOM

■

THE BRAIN BALANCE Program is the most comprehensive approach
to the treatment of autism, ADHD, Asperger's syndrome, dyslexia,
and the host of other neurobehavioral and neuroacademic disorders.
There is no other program like it in existence anywhere in the world.

It is a totally holistic program that has been proven to achieve measurable changes in behavior and academic performance. At best, it can permanently correct these disorders—meaning symptoms totally disappear.
At the least, symptoms will markedly diminish so that a child can resume
or begin to function in the real world, both socially and academically.

Brain Balance was revolutionary when we first started to use it in our
center more than fifteen years ago. It is now breaking new ground because
I have adapted our center program to one that can be used by a layperson
in a home setting. All it requires are commitment and the proper tools. I
will supply the tools but it is up to you to provide the commitment.

The Melillo At-Home Brain Balance Program takes the same unique
approach to rehabilitating the brain through what I call the three pillars
of brain development:

Sensory-motor exercises
Neuroacademic exercises
Bionutritional activities

The rest of this book is your workbook. In each of these three areas, you will do an assessment of your child that will identify if he has Functional Disconnection Syndrome and determine the type of imbalance he has. You will also learn how to assess your child's immune system for clues to the underlying source of his problem. And you will learn how to uncover well-hidden food intolerances that are exacerbating his symptoms and assess weaknesses in his digestive system.

I will then show you how to select a remediation program that encompasses the three pillars of brain development, develop a diet and supplement program, and even implement an effective behavior modification program that will put structure in your child's and your family's life.

You will be able to do all this with confidence. And you do not have to have a medical diagnosis to help guide you. Your confidence comes from having a complete understanding of what Brain Balance is all about, how it works, and most importantly, *why* it works. It is all summarized below in the Ten Principles of Brain Balance.

▪ Is Your Child a Candidate for Brain Balance? ▪

ANY child who has a learning or behavior problem that is not the result of physical damage to the brain can benefit from both the at-home or in-center Brain Balance Program.

Conditions that would exclude your child include but are not limited to organic brain diseases, Down syndrome, fragile X syndrome, infectious and metabolic diseases or injury, physical brain injury, strokes or brain tumors, psychiatric illness, personality disorders, or true behavioral disorders.

The Brain Balance Program works best with children who:

Can speak and can be responsive.
Have the ability to follow basic directions.
Are between the ages of four and seventeen years old.

Older children, however, must be motivated to change or you may not see dramatic positive results. It is difficult to make children over thirteen do something they don't want to do or if they don't believe they need any help. If this is the case, the child may need behavioral counseling or psychotherapy before trying this program. However, some of the most amazing results have been achieved on teenagers who are strongly motivated to change.

This home program is not a substitute for actual medical, psychiatric, or psychological treatment, and only a trained professional can make a medical diagnosis.

This book is not a substitute for professional treatment. It is also not a substitute for the Brain Balance Program in our centers, which is much more comprehensive and individualized to your child's needs. If you can afford or are located near a Brain Balance Center, we encourage you to enroll your child in that program. This home-based program is specifically designed to help assess and improve the balance and coordination of the brain and the body. ▪

Read through them carefully. Refer to them often. Absorb them. If they are not crystal clear, go back and reread Chapters 1 through 6.

THE TEN PRINCIPLES OF BRAIN BALANCE

Brain Balance and the success of implementing the program are based on these ten unique concepts:

1. **Childhood neurobehavioral and neuroacademic disorders are actually one condition with different sets of symptoms.** Brain Balance recognizes the majority of childhood neurological conditions as one disorder, Functional Disconnection Syndrome (FDS). Children display different symptoms depending on the part or parts of the brain affected.
2. **The underlying problem is a dysfunction in either the left or the right hemisphere that puts the brain out of sync.** All human functions are distributed in either the left or the right side of the brain, not both. To function properly, however, the brain must work as a whole. Symptoms of FDS differ depending on whether

the dysfunction is caused by a reduction of function, or an exaggeration of function in one hemisphere; or a reduction in function on one side and an exaggeration of function in the other.

3. **The problem and the dysfunctions must be accurately identified.** Brain Balance is specialized to assess, document, and objectively quantify Functional Disconnection Syndrome through the use of state-of-the-art testing in specific areas of function.

4. **The only way to correct the problem is to fix the imbalance, not treat the symptoms.** Fix the functional imbalance and the symptoms go away. Treat the symptoms with medication—the current and most popular approach—and brain function will never improve. Symptoms will return as soon as the medication wears off.

5. **All functional problems in the brain must be addressed individually.** If all the dysfunctions in the brain are not corrected, the symptoms will return and the problem will continue. Each function must be addressed one at a time.

6. **Success is achievable through a hemispheric-based program.** The only way to correct the imbalance is to stimulate the side of the brain that is out of balance without directly affecting the other side. Brain Balance uses a three-pronged program that includes sensory, motor, and academic exercises; behavioral techniques; and a nutritional program.

7. **Same Time Integration gets the brain back in sync.** The Brain Balance Program addresses each impaired function individually at first and gradually integrates exercises to achieve balance in the timing and rhythm between the left and the right sides of the brain. Same Time Integration incorporates all modalities simultaneously within the same time frame to get the left and the right brains working in synchronization.

8. **The brain and body must grow together.** Brain Balance is based on new science that shows that if the body is out of balance, the brain is out of balance, and vice versa to an equal degree.

9. **The problems are not primarily genetic and are therefore permanently correctable.** Brain Balance is based on the scientifically backed belief that the various symptoms of Functional Disconnection Syndrome are primarily the result of environmental factors. Genetic predisposition is the result of environmental fac-

tors that only alter the way a gene or genes are expressed. In other words, genes are not destiny.

10. **Parents play a crucial role in a child's individual success.** Parents have the power to achieve success using the Melillo At-Home Brain Balance Program. To this end, they must be motivated and fully involved in motivating their child to complete the required tasks. Correcting a behavior and/or learning disability through professional guidance and school involvement alone is not enough. However, using them in conjunction with the program can be a great help to parents and can even help enhance results.

Got it? Now you're ready to get started.

BRAIN BALANCE PROFILE: *Laura*

ASPERGER'S IS NOW A THING OF THE PAST

I first met Laura's mom when I gave a talk about learning disabilities to employees of a local SEPTA program in my town. She approached me afterward to tell me about her daughter.

Laura, she said, was a twelve-year-old whom doctors had diagnosed a few years ago with Asperger's syndrome, which is similar to and on the same spectrum as autism. Laura was bright and doing fine in school but she was a handful to deal and live with. Kids at school just considered her weird.

Laura, she said, stood out from kids in her class but not in a pleasant way. She shuffled rather than walked, always with her head slumped staring at her feet, and would stumble a lot. She was moody, never smiled, and rarely showed any expression. Her dad described her as downright mean.

Laura was sensitive to sound and touch. She wasn't into music like other kids because she couldn't stand the noise. Any loud noise—a train or cheers from a crowd at a ball game on TV (you could never take her to one!)—would make her cover her ears and grimace as if she were in pain. She couldn't stand the feeling of clothes against her body and always wore loose, baggy shirts and pants. "She's the only kid I know who doesn't wear jeans," lamented her mom.

While other little girls her age were experimenting with makeup and getting their ears pierced, Laura would have none of it. Most recently, Laura had stopped sleeping in her own bed and would only sleep on the family room couch—one more of Laura's many oddities that upset the family routines. I told Laura's mom about the Brain Balance Program and my belief that conditions such as autism and Asperger's are correctable, despite popular medical opinion to the contrary. Laura's mom seemed skeptical that we could help her. Nevertheless, she agreed to bring her in for an evaluation.

We noted things about Laura that no other specialists had ever mentioned. We pointed out that Laura had terrible spatial orientation, which was why she appeared so awkward and clumsy. She had very specific imbalances in her muscle tone and strength. And she was terrible when her eyes were closed, a classic sign of a right brain deficit. Her sensitivities and everything awkward about her were the result of slow growth in the right side of her brain that made it impossible to keep up with the left side. As a result, her ability to perform the skills regulated by the brain's right hemisphere were suppressed.

Convinced, Laura's parents enrolled her in our program. We started her on a daily after-school program of sensory, physical, and mental exercises as well as dietary changes.

Three weeks into the program, her mother was ecstatic over her progress. Not only was Laura now smiling and laughing more, she was actually becoming expressive. When someone pulled a practical joke on Laura's mom, Laura laughed and remarked, "Mom, you should have seen the expression on your face. It was so funny." Laura's mom was stunned. "She never used to notice the expression on anyone's face," her mom said. Laura was also sleeping in her own bed again.

From then on, Laura's whole world started to change. Kelly Clarkson was appearing in concert nearby and Laura asked if she could go. "Knowing she wanted to go to a concert—there'd be noise!—was exciting enough but I nearly dropped over when she picked out her clothes." Jeans (snug like the rest of the girls), jewelry (even dangly earrings), and makeup. Laura, she said, was so happy, she came home singing.

One day a few months later when they came to the clinic, Laura's mom called me aside. I could tell she was all excited about something. "Yesterday when I went to the bus stop to pick Laura up, I couldn't *find her. I didn't see her get off of the bus. I panicked, thinking something had happened to her. Then I saw her walking straight at me. I didn't even recognize my own daughter!" It was Laura—walking tall, head held high, laughing and talking in a group of girls. Her mom was crying tears of joy.*

When we retested Laura at the end of our formal program, the results proved what we suspected all along. She no longer had any signs of a right hemisphere weakness and her WIAT scores showed an evenness of left and right brain skills. Medical diagnostic testing revealed that she no longer met the criteria for a child with Asperger's or any disorder on the autism spectrum. To see Laura today, you could never imagine that she was once a child with "incurable" Asperger's syndrome.

7

MASTER HEMISPHERIC CHECKLIST

Identifying a Left or a Right Brain Deficiency

■

No amount of money would ever be enough for bringing such peace and normalcy to a family once living with chaos. This program has changed our lives.
There will never be enough words in this world to express what is in my heart.

—DORIS, MOTHER OF SIX-YEAR-OLD SEAN,
WHO WAS DIAGNOSED WITH AUTISM

■

THIS MASTER CHECKLIST contains all the characteristics of a child
with Functional Disconnection Syndrome and is a key tool that you
will use through the Brain Balance Program. There are 200 characteristics—100 signify a right brain deficit and 100 signify a left brain deficit. This
checklist will help you determine if your child has FDS and which side of
the brain is causing it. The greater the number of checkmarks, the more
severe the imbalance, and the longer it may take for your child to achieve
a natural balance. (Checklists in Chapter 8 will help you more specifically
determine which function or functions in the brain are weakest.)

You will also use this checklist to help measure your child's progress.
You can use it at any time. In fact, it is a good idea to check back with it
periodically after the program is completed to make sure that your child
is not regressing.

Go through the checklist for the first time before you begin the assessment part of the program that begins in Chapter 8 and at the recommended intervals suggested here. Feel free to go back to this list anytime
you feel it is necessary. Remember when you answer these questions, your

answers should be based on a comparison with typically developing children the same age. Also if your child is on medication, answer based on how the child would compare when not on the medication.

MOTOR CHARACTERISTICS OF A RIGHT BRAIN DELAY

	Start of Program	4 wks	8 wks	12 wks
☐ Clumsiness and an odd posture	☐	☐	☐	☐
☐ Poor coordination				
☐ Not athletically inclined and has no interest in popular childhood participation sports	☐	☐	☐	☐
☐ Low muscle tone—muscles seem kind of floppy	☐	☐	☐	☐
☐ Poor gross motor skills, such as difficulty learning to ride a bike and/or runs and/or walks oddly	☐	☐	☐	☐
☐ Repetitive/stereotyped motor mannerisms (spins in circles, flaps arms)	☐	☐	☐	☐
☐ Fidgets excessively	☐	☐	☐	☐
☐ Poor eye contact	☐	☐	☐	☐
☐ Walks or walked on toes when younger	☐	☐	☐	☐

Total _____

MOTOR CHARACTERISTICS OF A LEFT BRAIN DELAY

	Start of Program	4 wks	8 wks	12 wks
☐ Fine motor problems (poor or slow handwriting)	☐	☐	☐	☐
☐ Difficulty with fine motor skills, such as buttoning a shirt	☐	☐	☐	☐
☐ Poor or immature hand grip when writing	☐	☐	☐	☐
☐ Tends to write very large for age or grade level	☐	☐	☐	☐
☐ Stumbles over words when fatigued	☐	☐	☐	☐
☐ Exhibited delay in crawling, standing, and/or walking	☐	☐	☐	☐
☐ Loves sports and is good at them	☐	☐	☐	☐
☐ Good muscle tone	☐	☐	☐	☐

continued

	Start of Program	4 wks	8 wks	12 wks
☐ Poor drawing skills	☐	☐	☐	☐
☐ Difficulty learning to play music	☐	☐	☐	☐
☐ Likes to fix things with the hands and is interested in anything mechanical	☐	☐	☐	☐
☐ Difficulty planning and coordinating body movements	☐	☐	☐	☐

Total _____

SENSORY CHARACTERISTICS OF A RIGHT BRAIN DELAY

	Start of Program	4 wks	8 wks	12 wks
☐ Poor spatial orientation—bumps into things often	☐	☐	☐	☐
☐ Sensitivity to sound	☐	☐	☐	☐
☐ Confusion when asked to point to different body parts	☐	☐	☐	☐
☐ Poor sense of balance	☐	☐	☐	☐
☐ High threshold for pain—doesn't cry when gets a cut	☐	☐	☐	☐
☐ Likes to spin, go on rides, swing, etc.—anything with motion	☐	☐	☐	☐
☐ Touches things compulsively	☐	☐	☐	☐
☐ A girl uninterested in makeup or jewelry	☐	☐	☐	☐
☐ Does not like the feel of clothing on arms or legs; pulls off clothes	☐	☐	☐	☐
☐ Doesn't like being touched and doesn't like to touch things	☐	☐	☐	☐
☐ Incessantly smells everything	☐	☐	☐	☐
☐ Prefers bland foods	☐	☐	☐	☐
☐ Does not notice strong smells, such as burning wood, popcorn, or cookies baking in the oven	☐	☐	☐	☐
☐ Avoids food because of the way it looks	☐	☐	☐	☐
☐ Hates having to eat and is not even interested in sweets	☐	☐	☐	☐
☐ Extremely picky eater	☐	☐	☐	☐

Total _____

SENSORY CHARACTERISTICS OF A LEFT BRAIN DELAY

	Start of Program	4 wks	8 wks	12 wks
Doesn't seem to have many sensory issues or problems, such as a sensitivity to sound	☐	☐	☐	☐
Has good spatial awareness	☐	☐	☐	☐
Has good sense of balance	☐	☐	☐	☐
Eats just about anything	☐	☐	☐	☐
Has a normal to above-average sense of taste and smell	☐	☐	☐	☐
Likes to be hugged and held	☐	☐	☐	☐
Does not have any oddities concerning clothing	☐	☐	☐	☐
Has auditory processing problems	☐	☐	☐	☐
Seems not to hear well, although hearing tests normal	☐	☐	☐	☐
Delay in speaking was attributed to ear infections	☐	☐	☐	☐
Gets motion sick and has other motion sickness issues	☐	☐	☐	☐
Is not undersensitive or oversensitive to pain	☐	☐	☐	☐

Total _____

EMOTIONAL CHARACTERISTICS OF A RIGHT BRAIN DEFICIENCY

	Start of Program	4 wks	8 wks	12 wks
Spontaneously cries and/or laughs and has sudden outbursts of anger or fear	☐	☐	☐	☐
Worries a lot and has several phobias	☐	☐	☐	☐
Holds on to past "hurts"	☐	☐	☐	☐
Has sudden emotional outbursts that appear overreactive and inappropriate to the situation	☐	☐	☐	☐
Experiences panic and/or anxiety attacks	☐	☐	☐	☐
Sometimes displays dark or violent thoughts	☐	☐	☐	☐
Face lacks expression; doesn't exhibit much body language	☐	☐	☐	☐
Too uptight; cannot seem to loosen up	☐	☐	☐	☐
Lacks empathy and feelings for others	☐	☐	☐	☐

continued

	Start of Program	4 wks	8 wks	12 wks
☐ Lacks emotional reciprocity	☐	☐	☐	☐
☐ Often seems fearless and is a risk taker	☐	☐	☐	☐

Total _____

EMOTIONAL CHARACTERISTICS OF A LEFT BRAIN DEFICIENCY

	Start of Program	4 wks	8 wks	12 wks
☐ Overly happy and affectionate; loves to hug and kiss	☐	☐	☐	☐
☐ Frequently moody and irritable	☐	☐	☐	☐
☐ Loves doing new or different things but gets bored easily	☐	☐	☐	☐
☐ Lacks motivation	☐	☐	☐	☐
☐ Withdrawn and shy	☐	☐	☐	☐
☐ Excessively cautious, pessimistic, or negative	☐	☐	☐	☐
☐ Doesn't seem to get any pleasure out of life	☐	☐	☐	☐
☐ Socially withdrawn	☐	☐	☐	☐
☐ Cries easily; feelings get hurt easily	☐	☐	☐	☐
☐ Seems to be in touch with own feelings	☐	☐	☐	☐
☐ Empathetic to other people's feelings; reads people's emotions well	☐	☐	☐	☐
☐ Gets embarrassed easily	☐	☐	☐	☐
☐ Very sensitive to what others think about him or her	☐	☐	☐	☐

Total _____

BEHAVIORAL CHARACTERISTICS OF A RIGHT BRAIN DELAY

	Start of Program	4 wks	8 wks	12 wks
☐ Logical thinker	☐	☐	☐	☐
☐ Often misses the gist of a story	☐	☐	☐	☐
☐ Always the last to get a joke	☐	☐	☐	☐
☐ Gets stuck in set behavior; can't let it go	☐	☐	☐	☐
☐ Lacks social tact and/or is antisocial and/or socially isolated	☐	☐	☐	☐

	Start of Program	4 wks	8 wks	12 wks
Poor time management; is always late	☐	☐	☐	☐
Disorganized	☐	☐	☐	☐
Has a problem paying attention	☐	☐	☐	☐
Is hyperactive and/or impulsive	☐	☐	☐	☐
Has obsessive thoughts or behaviors	☐	☐	☐	☐
Argues all the time and is generally uncooperative	☐	☐	☐	☐
Exhibits signs of an eating disorder	☐	☐	☐	☐
Failed to thrive as an infant	☐	☐	☐	☐
Mimics sounds or words repeatedly without really understanding the meaning	☐	☐	☐	☐
Appears bored, aloof, and abrupt	☐	☐	☐	☐
Considered strange by other children	☐	☐	☐	☐
Inability to form friendships	☐	☐	☐	☐
Has difficulty sharing enjoyment, interests, or achievements with other people	☐	☐	☐	☐
Inappropriately giddy or silly	☐	☐	☐	☐
Acts inappropriately in social situations	☐	☐	☐	☐
Talks incessantly and asks the same question repetitively	☐	☐	☐	☐
Has no or little joint attention, such as the need to point to an object to get your attention	☐	☐	☐	☐
Didn't look at self in mirror as a toddler	☐	☐	☐	☐

Total _____

BEHAVIORAL CHARACTERISTICS OF A LEFT BRAIN DELAY

	Start of Program	4 wks	8 wks	12 wks
Procrastinates	☐	☐	☐	☐
Is extremely shy, especially around strangers	☐	☐	☐	☐
Is very good at nonverbal communication	☐	☐	☐	☐
Is well liked by other children and teachers	☐	☐	☐	☐
Does not have any behavioral problems in school	☐	☐	☐	☐
Understands social rules	☐	☐	☐	☐
Has poor self-esteem	☐	☐	☐	☐
Hates doing homework	☐	☐	☐	☐

continued

	Start of Program	4 wks	8 wks	12 wks
☐ Is very good at social interaction	☐	☐	☐	☐
☐ Makes good eye contact	☐	☐	☐	☐
☐ Likes to be around people and enjoys social activities, such as going to parties	☐	☐	☐	☐
☐ Doesn't like to go to sleepovers	☐	☐	☐	☐
☐ Is not good at following routines	☐	☐	☐	☐
☐ Can't follow multiple-step directions	☐	☐	☐	☐
☐ Is in touch with own feelings	☐	☐	☐	☐
☐ Jumps to conclusions	☐	☐	☐	☐

Total _____

ACADEMIC CHARACTERISTICS OF A RIGHT BRAIN DELAY

	Start of Program	4 wks	8 wks	12 wks
☐ Poor math reasoning (word problems, geometry, algebra)	☐	☐	☐	☐
☐ Poor reading comprehension and pragmatic skills	☐	☐	☐	☐
☐ Misses the big picture	☐	☐	☐	☐
☐ Very analytical	☐	☐	☐	☐
☐ Likes "slapstick" or obvious physical humor	☐	☐	☐	☐
☐ Is very good at finding mistakes (spelling)	☐	☐	☐	☐
☐ Takes everything literally	☐	☐	☐	☐
☐ Doesn't always reach a conclusion when speaking	☐	☐	☐	☐
☐ Started speaking early	☐	☐	☐	☐
☐ Has tested for a high IQ, but scores run the whole spectrum; or IQ is above normal in verbal ability and below average in performance abilities	☐	☐	☐	☐
☐ Was an early word reader	☐	☐	☐	☐
☐ Is interested in unusual topics	☐	☐	☐	☐
☐ Learns in a rote (memorizing) manner	☐	☐	☐	☐
☐ Learns extraordinary amounts of specific facts about a subject	☐	☐	☐	☐
☐ Is impatient	☐	☐	☐	☐
☐ Speaks in a monotone; has little voice inflection	☐	☐	☐	☐

	Start of Program	4 wks	8 wks	12 wks
☐ Is a poor nonverbal communicator	☐	☐	☐	☐
☐ Doesn't like loud noises (like fireworks)	☐	☐	☐	☐
☐ Speaks out loud regarding what he or she is thinking	☐	☐	☐	☐
☐ Talks "in your face"—is a space invader	☐	☐	☐	☐
☐ Good reader but does not enjoy reading	☐	☐	☐	☐
☐ Analytical; led by logic	☐	☐	☐	☐
☐ Follows rules without questioning them	☐	☐	☐	☐
☐ Good at keeping track of time	☐	☐	☐	☐
☐ Easily memorizes spelling and mathematical formulas	☐	☐	☐	☐
☐ Enjoys observing rather than participating	☐	☐	☐	☐
☐ Would rather read an instruction manual before trying something new	☐	☐	☐	☐
☐ Math was often the first academic subject that became a problem	☐	☐	☐	☐

Total _____

ACADEMIC CHARACTERISTICS OF A LEFT BRAIN DELAY

	Start of Program	4 wks	8 wks	12 wks
☐ Very good at big picture skills	☐	☐	☐	☐
☐ Is an intuitive thinker and is led by feelings	☐	☐	☐	☐
☐ Good at abstract "free" association	☐	☐	☐	☐
☐ Poor analytical skills	☐	☐	☐	☐
☐ Very visual; loves images and patterns	☐	☐	☐	☐
☐ Constantly questions why you're doing something or why rules exist	☐	☐	☐	☐
☐ Has poor sense of time	☐	☐	☐	☐
☐ Enjoys touching and feeling actual objects	☐	☐	☐	☐
☐ Has trouble prioritizing	☐	☐	☐	☐
☐ Is unlikely to read instructions before trying something new	☐	☐	☐	☐
☐ Is naturally creative, but needs to work hard to develop full potential	☐	☐	☐	☐

continued

		Start of Program	4 wks	8 wks	12 wks
☐	Would rather do things instead of observe	☐	☐	☐	☐
☐	Uses good voice inflection when speaking	☐	☐	☐	☐
☐	Misreads or omits common small words	☐	☐	☐	☐
☐	Has difficulty saying long words	☐	☐	☐	☐
☐	Reads very slowly and laboriously	☐	☐	☐	☐
☐	Had difficulty naming colors, objects, and letters as a toddler	☐	☐	☐	☐
☐	Needs to hear or see concepts many times in order to learn them	☐	☐	☐	☐
☐	Has shown a downward trend in achievement test scores or school performance	☐	☐	☐	☐
☐	Schoolwork is inconsistent	☐	☐	☐	☐
☐	Was a late talker	☐	☐	☐	☐
☐	Has difficulty pronouncing words (poor with phonics)	☐	☐	☐	☐
☐	Had difficulty learning the alphabet, nursery rhymes, or songs when young	☐	☐	☐	☐
☐	Has difficulty finishing homework or finishing a conversation	☐	☐	☐	☐
☐	Acts before thinking and makes careless mistakes	☐	☐	☐	☐
☐	Daydreams a lot	☐	☐	☐	☐
☐	Has difficulty sequencing events in the proper order	☐	☐	☐	☐
☐	Often writes letters backward	☐	☐	☐	☐
☐	Is poor at basic math skills	☐	☐	☐	☐
☐	Has poor memorization skills	☐	☐	☐	☐
☐	Has poor academic ability	☐	☐	☐	☐
☐	Has an IQ lower than expected and verbal scores are lower than nonverbal scores	☐	☐	☐	☐
☐	Performs poorly on verbal tests	☐	☐	☐	☐
☐	Needs to be told to do something several times before acting on it	☐	☐	☐	☐
☐	Stutters or stuttered when younger	☐	☐	☐	☐
☐	Is a poor speller	☐	☐	☐	☐
☐	Doesn't read directions well	☐	☐	☐	☐

Total _____

COMMON IMMUNE CHARACTERISTICS OF A RIGHT BRAIN DELAY

	Start of Program	4 wks	8 wks	12 wks
Has lots of allergies	☐	☐	☐	☐
Rarely gets colds and infections	☐	☐	☐	☐
Has had or has eczema or asthma	☐	☐	☐	☐
Skin has little white bumps, especially on the back of the arms	☐	☐	☐	☐
Displays erratic behavior—good one day, bad the next	☐	☐	☐	☐
Craves certain foods, especially dairy and wheat products	☐	☐	☐	☐

Total _____

COMMON IMMUNE CHARACTERISTICS OF A LEFT BRAIN DELAY

	Start of Program	4 wks	8 wks	12 wks
Gets chronic ear infections	☐	☐	☐	☐
Prone to benign tumors or cysts	☐	☐	☐	☐
Has taken antibiotics more than ten to fifteen times before the age of ten	☐	☐	☐	☐
Has had tubes put in the ears	☐	☐	☐	☐
Catches colds frequently	☐	☐	☐	☐
No allergies	☐	☐	☐	☐

Total _____

AUTONOMIC CHARACTERISTICS OF A RIGHT BRAIN DELAY

	Start of Program	4 wks	8 wks	12 wks
Problems with bowels, such as constipation and diarrhea	☐	☐	☐	☐
Has a rapid heart rate and/or high blood pressure for age	☐	☐	☐	☐
Appears bloated, especially after meals, and often complains of stomach pains	☐	☐	☐	☐
Has body odor	☐	☐	☐	☐

continued

	Start of Program	4 wks	8 wks	12 wks
☐ Sweats a lot	☐	☐	☐	☐
☐ Hands are always moist and clammy	☐	☐	☐	☐

Total _____

AUTONOMIC CHARACTERISTICS OF A LEFT BRAIN DELAY

	Start of Program	4 wks	8 wks	12 wks
☐ Has a bedwetting problem	☐	☐	☐	☐
☐ Has or had an irregular heartbeat, such as an arrhythmia or a heart murmur	☐	☐	☐	☐

Total _____

TAKING THE TOTAL

Here count up the total checks you've made for left brain and right brain symptoms.

Right brain total _____
Left brain total _____
Grand total _____

There are a total of 200 characteristics in this master checklist. The total number of checks that you have made can give you an overall idea as to the severity of the problem as a whole. However, the main finding is simply whether there are more checks on one side than the other.

The general guideline of severity is based on the total number of checks on both sides combined, as follows:

Mild—50 or below
Moderate—50 to 100
Severe—100 or above

This should be considered with the level of the imbalance, meaning the greater the difference in the two totals, the greater the imbalance, and the more time it may take to correct. Remember, the weak hemisphere is the side with the most checks.

Hemispheric weakness is on the _____ side of the brain.

❧ BRAIN BALANCE PROFILE: *Brian*

LIKE A NEW LITTLE PERSON

When Brian and his mom first came to Brain Balance, it was quite obvious that he'd had a trying young life. He'd been born four years earlier after an induced labor and complicated delivery. His mom said he seemed frail almost from the day he was born.

Since he was her third child, Brian's mom was able to recognize that his development didn't seem to be going right. He had a pronounced head tilt that was attended to by a physical therapist. He had been delayed in crawling and walking and his mom described his crawl as quite different from his siblings. Then around the age of eighteen months, his development seemed to come to a halt. As his mother described, his language didn't grow and he "began to tune out the world around him." He was diagnosed with severe autism.

When Brian came to Brain Balance, he was not toilet trained, couldn't dress himself, and wouldn't make eye contact. He barely spoke and was afraid of things that gave other kids a thrill, like swinging and playing on a jungle gym. He was remote, even around his parents. Testing showed that he was nutritionally deficient, which was no surprise considering the fact that his diet was limited to only the few foods he would eat. So, we modeled a supplement program that addressed his many deficiencies.

After two weeks on Brain Balance, he finally "got it" and was toilet trained. He was also sleeping better. After twelve weeks, he was like a new little person. Where at the start he would only utter a few words, he was now expressive and talkative. He was looking at people and greeting them. And, his mom reported, she was taking him to the playground. "He wants to swing as high as he possibly can go," she reported. Not only that, Brian started to dress himself and showed an interest in trying new foods. For such a young boy with an unusual number of issues, he was 75 percent on his way to recovery.

8

HEMISPHERIC HOME SENSORY-MOTOR ASSESSMENT

How to Detect a Left or a Right Brain Deficiency

■

Christian would not be making the amazing strides that he is, both academically and socially. It's like he loves life again. I always knew what an amazing, outgoing, funny, smart, gentle, loving kid he was, but now everyone is seeing it and commenting on it.

—KRISTEN M., CHRISTIAN'S MOM

■

You are now armed with the essential information you need to start the Melillo At-Home Brain Balance Program. You understand that Functional Disconnection Syndrome is an umbrella label for the whole spectrum of behavior and learning disabilities resulting from an imbalance in the developing brain and that the symptoms vary depending on the side of the brain that is growing too slow or too fast.

You also know that this is not a disease in which the brain is damaged. It's an environmentally caused dysfunction that can be corrected through sensory-motor and academic exercises and a change in diet. These exercises must be tailored to the specific dysfunction in the dysfunctional hemisphere. Identifying the hemisphere and the areas of dysfunction is the first—and most crucial—step to getting the brain in rhythm and reconnecting the brain of your Disconnected Child. That is what you are going to do now. These assessment tests and checklists are going to lead you to identifying if your child has a right brain imbalance or a left brain imbalance. I will then show you how to use this information to tailor a program of exercises that begins in the next chapter.

YOUR ASSESSMENT BRIEFING

Each hemisphere has separate circuits and centers that control various sensory and motor functions. What you will be doing is isolating the specific functions that are the weakest. As you do the assessment tests, it will become obvious that your child's strong functions are specific to one side of the brain and his or her weakest functions are specific to the opposite side.

You will be assessing your child in ten areas:

Mother and Child Health History
Developmental Milestones History
Sensory-Motor Skills
Left Side, Right Side Dominance
Vestibular (Balance) Skills
Auditory (Hearing) Skills
Vision Skills
Proprioception Skills
Tactile (Touch) Skills
Olfactory (Smell and Taste) Skills

Prior to starting most of these assessments, you will fill out a ten-question checklist and rate your child on a scale of 1 to 10. A 1 means "does not apply," a 5 is "this sounds somewhat" like my child, and a 10 is "almost always"—this sounds exactly like my child.

After you've completed all the checklists and assessments, I will show you how to tally them up and determine if your child has a left brain or a right brain deficiency. Then I will teach you how to correct it.

BASIC RULES

You should not attempt to do these assessments all in one day. Do them over the course of three to four days, or even a week. Review and fill out the checklist before you do each assessment. It is important that you answer these questions accurately, so consult with others—teachers, day care workers, babysitters, whoever is necessary. The tests can be done with only one parent participating. However, it is best for both parents to confer and agree on the answers.

If both parents want to be involved, fill them out separately then compare notes. It is important that you and the child be in the right frame of mind. For example, if you're in a bad mood or your child is being fussy, then postpone the assessment to another time.

Most children with FDS are very bright, so you want to explain everything you are doing but not necessarily the reason you are doing it—that is, you don't want to say you are trying to find out what is wrong with him or her. Rather, make it appear more like a game. I've done these assessments with children thousands of times, and for the most part, they really enjoy them and will get engaged as long as they feel like it is fun and they do not feel threatened. Do not comment on what you are seeing or discovering. Encourage your child all the time and give a lot of positive feedback. If the child seems uncomfortable or scared at any time, stop. You can always redo the test at another time. Most likely, your child will enjoy all the attention and like spending the time with you.

Do the assessments in a location that is familiar to the child and is also comfortable, quiet, away from distraction, and has plenty of light. If your child is sensitive to light, make sure to adjust for it.

For these tests you will need certain tools, which you should make sure you have, borrow, or purchase before you begin. These tools are:

Penlight or small flashlight
Tuning fork, preferably a C-128
Two small unused paintbrushes
A straight chair
A chair with arms that spins around
A mat or soft surface for lying on the floor
Several empty film canisters
Essential oils of aromas familiar to your child, such as orange or
    lemon

Some children may be too small or too low-functioning to do these assessments. It is also possible that some of the results you get will not be very clear or you may not be able to determine a specific level. In these instances you can depend on the results you get from the symptoms checklist in each section. At the end I will show you how to use the symptom checklists along with the Master Hemispheric Checklist to determine the side and level of dysfunction in each sensory and motor area.

Each sensory-motor test is broken down, when possible, to three functional levels:

Level 1: the lowest functional level
Level 2: mid-level
Level 3: the highest functional level (this is the ultimate goal)

Here is one other important message before you begin. These checklists and assessments do not constitute a formal neurological or physical exam, or a professional diagnosis. This can only be done by a professional. These checklists and assessments are simply a guide to help you evaluate your child.

If you find this difficult or your child does not respond, then you may need a more complete professional evaluation and/or your child would benefit best from an individualized program, such as we provide at a Brain Balance Center. You should try to find a local Brain Balance Center or a professional who has been trained in Hemispheric Integration Therapy or Functional Neurology.

ABOUT THE ASSESSMENTS

You will begin developing your corrective home program by evaluating your child's sensory-motor functions. Sensory-motor activities, which you will get to in the next chapter, form the most important part of the Brain Balance Program.

As you now know, the foundation of baseline brain activity and balance comes from sensory and motor stimulation to the brain. Also, the most common symptoms that we see in children with FDS involve the muscles—lack of coordination, low muscle tone, clumsiness, bad posture, an awkward gait, and so on. Sensory stimulation is what drives brain development and activity, but it is the motor system that drives the sensory system.

I have never seen a child who has just one sensory deficit, so you should not be looking for just one. Likewise, we never see a child with only gross (large muscle) or fine (small muscle) motor problems. It is usually a combination of both, although they usually have more of a problem with one or the other.

In addition, it is impossible, unless the child has a specific brain injury, to have sensory deficits without various emotional, cognitive, immune, autonomic, and academic issues. However, the combination of these problems is different in each child. This is why these evaluations are so important. Relying on a list of symptoms alone is not the best way to identify what your child's specific problems are, or what activities the child must do to resolve these problems. Symptoms can be misleading but functions don't lie.

Before you start, however, I want you to go back in time and review some things that will help you understand how your child got to this point.

MOTHER AND CHILD HEALTH HISTORY

Studies show a link between learning and behavior disorders and the early health history of either mother or child. Signs of a brain deficiency can show up early—in some children even before they are born. This is especially true of a right brain deficiency. Many clues can be found when looking back at your child's development history and your own health history and pregnancy—go through these lists. You don't have to write anything down or keep a tally. It is just one more assessment that will help you determine if your child has FDS and if it is due to a left or a right brain delay.

▶ *Mother's Health Profile*

PREGNANCY
Difficulty getting pregnant, one or more miscarriages, or complications during pregnancies
Fertility drug use

PRENATAL
History of allergies and immune deficiencies, chronic fatigue, or fibromyalgia
Gestational diabetes

Thyroid dysfunction and possibly exposed to toxic chemicals or
   pesticides

BIRTH
Breech presentation
Forceps delivery
Oxygen deprivation
Bruising or swelling about head and neck
Induced labor

BIRTH TO AGE ONE
Colic and other digestive problems
Alternate chronic constipation and diarrhea
Spitting up (reflux) or projectile vomiting
Pyloric stenosis (stomach obstruction)
Allergies and/or asthma
Thrush (yeast infection)
Eczema at birth that got worse
Chronic ear infections that were aggressively treated with
   antibiotics
Reactions to immunization
Sleep disturbances
Hypotonia (low muscle tone)
Possible sensory deprivation prior to adoption

AGES ONE TO TWO
Allergic symptoms: constant runny nose, red ears, puffy eyes
White bumps on skin
Increasing hyperactivity
Strabismus (lazy eye), possibly nystagmus (involuntary shaking
   of the eyes side to side)
Regression in milestones around age two

DIET
Increasing limited diet due to strong likes and dislikes
Preference for foods containing wheat and dairy
Preference for milk and cereal or a bagel with cream cheese for
   breakfast

Preference for grilled cheese sandwiches for lunch
Preference for pizza or pasta for dinner or secondarily chicken
    nuggets
Snacks on raw carrots
Loves eating French fries

AGES TWO TO THREE
Delayed or abnormal crawling, or skipped stages of crawling
    before walking
Clumsy or floppy movements
Toe-in foot or knock-kneed
Lisp in speech

▶ Normal Vital Signs

As the child grows, the first areas of the brain that develop are those that control reflexes. An area called the medulla controls the automatic reflexes, such as breathing and heartbeat, that are necessary for basic survival.

That's why they are called vital signs. There are basic values for heart rate, breathing rate, and blood pressure as a child matures. When a child is first born, the heart rate and respiratory rate are very rapid and blood pressure is relatively high. As higher areas of the brain develop, heart rate and breathing slow down and blood pressure drops. Once a child starts to stand and walk, heart rate and respiration get slower.

If your child's brain is progressing normally, heart rate, respiratory rate, and blood pressure should match what is considered normal for certain age levels. By age three, the cerebral cortex should be taking over and inhibiting the primitive system that has been supporting vital functions since birth. If it is still too rapid at age three, it is an indication that the brain is immature for his or her chronological age. Some parents keep baby books that call for these entries. If you don't have one, ask your pediatrician's office to get you a copy. Compare them to this table.

Age	Avg. Heart Rate	Avg. Respiratory Rate	Avg. Blood Pressure
Newborn	140	30–75	
1–6 months	130		
6–12 months	115	22–31	
1–2 years	110	17–23	96/60–112/78 (2 yrs)

Age	Avg. Heart Rate	Avg. Respiratory Rate	Avg. Blood Pressure
2–6 years	103	16–25 (2–4 yrs)	98/64–116/80 (6 yrs)
6–10 years	95	13–23 (4–10 yrs)	106/68–126/84 (9 yrs)
10–14 years	85	13–19	
14–18 years	82	same as adult	112/74–136/88 (12 yrs)

Most likely you'll find that your child's record is off the chart. Most likely it still is. Brain Balance can improve this.

Throughout the program you will keep track of your child's heart rate, breathing rate, and blood pressure. Do this once a week if possible. You can start tracking it now. Take your child's heart rate by counting the beats per minute at the wrist. You can easily measure their breathing rate by watching and recording how often your child's chest rises and falls in a ten-second period then multiply that by 6 to get their breaths per minute. You must do this when the child is not aware of it. Ask your pediatrician to check your child's blood pressure on both arms (they should be relatively equal). If there is a significant difference (more than 10 points) in any of the numbers, this is usually caused by a brain imbalance. The higher number is usually on the same side as the weaker hemisphere. As your child progresses through the program, you will see a change in vital signs.

DEVELOPMENTAL MILESTONES ASSESSMENT

During the first year of life, a baby grows at an amazing speed. Weight doubles by five or six months and triples by the first birthday. A baby is constantly learning. Major achievements, called developmental milestones, include rolling over, sitting up, standing, walking, and saying those first words. No two children are exactly alike. Most babies reach certain milestones at similar ages. However, it's not unusual for a healthy, "normal" baby to fall behind in some areas or race ahead in others. If your child was born prematurely (before thirty-seven weeks of pregnancy), you need to look at the milestone guidelines a little differently. The age at which a child is expected to reach various milestones is based on the due date, not the birthday. So if your child was born two months early, then you should add two months to each milestone. Compare your child's development to the table below. Make note if your child was early or late. Either one can be a sign that a child's underlying problem may have existed at birth. Again you don't have to write anything down or keep a tally.

This table is the standard used by the American Academy of Pediatrics. I have found, however, that the real time frames are much shorter. For instance, according to the AAP, it is considered normal for a child to start walking between eleven and sixteen months of age. However, I have found that if the child starts to walk after thirteen or fourteen months, it is a sign of developmental delay.

Many parents are delighted to see their child walk earlier than expected. They see it as a good sign. This isn't necessarily the case. I have found that if a child starts to walk before ten or eleven months, it is also a sign of a developmental problem. In order for the nervous system to develop properly, a child must crawl for at least two to four months before starting to walk.

▼ **HINT:** In my experience, most parents are excellent at remembering if their child was early or missed a major milestone. If you can't remember some of these details, it is probably because there was nothing out of the ordinary.

▶ Milestones

By the end of their first month, most babies:

Make jerky, quivering arm movements
Bring hands near face
Keep hands in tight fists
Move head from side to side while lying on stomach
Focus on objects 8 to 12 inches away
Prefer human faces over other shapes
Prefer black-and-white or high-contrast patterns
Hear very well
Recognize some sounds, including parents' voices

By the end of their third month, most babies:

Raise head and chest when lying on stomach
Support upper body with arms when lying on stomach
Stretch legs out and kick when lying on stomach or back

Push down on legs when feet are placed on a firm surface
Open and shut hands
Bring hands to mouth
Grab and shake hand toys
Follow moving object with eyes
Watch faces closely
Recognize familiar objects and people at a distance
Start using hands and eyes in coordination
Begin to babble and to imitate some sounds
Smile at the sound of parents' voices
Enjoy playing with other people
May cry when playing stops

By the end of their seventh month, most babies:

Roll over both ways (stomach to back and back to stomach)
Sit up
Reach for object with hand
Transfer objects from one hand to the other
Support whole weight on legs when held upright
Develop full-color vision and mature distance vision
Use voice to express joy and displeasure
Respond to own name
Babble chains of consonants (ba-ba-ba-ba)
Distinguish emotions by tone of voice
Explore objects with hands and mouth
Struggle to get objects that are out of reach
Enjoy playing peek-a-boo
Show an interest in mirror images
Crawl

By their first birthday, most babies:

Sit without assistance
Get into hands-and-knees position
Pull self up to stand
Walk holding on to furniture, and possibly a few steps without
    support

Use pincer grasp (thumb and forefinger)

Say "dada" and "mama"

Use exclamations, such as "uh-oh!"

Try to imitate words

Respond to "no" and simple verbal requests

Use simple gestures, such as shaking head "no" and waving bye-bye

Explore objects in many ways (shaking, banging, throwing, dropping)

Begin to use objects correctly (drinking from cup, brushing hair)

Find hidden objects easily

Look at correct picture when an image is named

By their second birthday, most children:

Walk alone

Pull toys behind them while walking

Carry large toy or several toys while walking

Begin to run

Kick a ball

Climb on and off furniture without help

Walk up and down stairs while holding on to support

Scribble with crayon

Build tower of four blocks or more

Recognize names of familiar people, objects, and body parts

Say several single words (by fifteen to eighteen months)

Use simple phrases (by eighteen to twenty-four months)

Use two- to four-word sentences ("want snack")

Follow simple instructions

Begin to sort objects by shapes and colors

Begin to play make-believe

Imitate behavior of others

Show growing independence

Source: Adapted from American Academy of Pediatrics, *Caring for Your Baby and Young Child: Birth to Age 5*, Fourth Edition (Bantam Books, 2005).

·   ·   ·

MIXED DOMINANCE ASSESSMENT

Ideally, children should have a dominant side when it comes to using their hand, foot, eye, and ear. If they do not, it most often is a sign that the brain is not developing or maturing properly. A child's mixed dominance can be changed and the natural dominance released through the Brain Balance Program. We see it happen all the time. This does not mean that all children who are left-handed should be right-handed, but they should favor one side from head to toe. Here is how to find out.

Here you will be determining your child's laterality. You are checking to find out if he favors left or right for:

Hand
Foot
Eye
Ear

If you find that your child's dominance is mixed, repeat this test each week, as you go through the Brain Balance Program. Seeing a change is a good sign, but it doesn't have to happen in all children.

▶ *Hand*

You likely already know if your child is left- or right-handed, but do this test anyway. Record your finding in the space provided. Do this test outdoors.

Find a ball, such as a baseball, that is small enough for your child to catch with one hand. Stand a few feet away from your child and start tossing the ball back and forth. Little kids have a tendency to play catch with two hands, so you'll have to instruct your child to try to catch it with only one hand.

Hand used _____

Which hand does the child use to draw, crayon, or write?

Hand used _____

Which hand does the child use to brush her teeth?

Hand used _____

Ask the child if he is left-handed, right-handed, or has mixed dominance. The answer is:

_____

▶ *Foot*

This exercise will tell you which foot is dominant, as foot preference is not something that is taught, such as handwriting in which a child is often urged to use the right hand. Ask the child to kick a very light ball across the room. If this is not available, bunch up some newspaper into a ball. Do this three times.

1. L_____ R_____
2. L_____ R_____
3. L_____ R_____

Ask the child to take off her shoes and, while standing, write her name on the floor with her toes. She doesn't have to actually finish this task. You want to find out which foot she uses. Do this on three different occasions.

1. L_____ R_____
2. L_____ R_____
3. L_____ R_____

▶ *Eye*

NEAR VISION

Hand the child a kaleidoscope or magnifying glass and ask him to look through it. Which eye does he use?

R_____ L_____

• • •

FAR VISION

Take a tube, such as one from a roll of paper towels. Select a small stationary object, such as a doorknob or light switch, and ask the child to focus on the object with one eye by looking through the tube. Hand the child the tube, pointing it at the center of his body. Tell him to take the tube with both hands, hold it at arm's length, and slowly bring it toward the eye. Note which eye he uses to focus on the object.

Do this three times with three different objects. Make sure that you aim at the center of the body when you hand the tube to the child and that the child grasps it with both hands before you let it go.

Object 1. R _____ L _____
Object 2. R _____ L _____
Object 3. R _____ L _____

▶ *Ear*

Ideally you should use a tuning fork for this test. A C-128 is preferable. Demonstrate this task first before asking the child to do it. Make sure you turn your head and put one ear to the tuning fork when demonstrating. If you don't have a tuning fork, you can use a cell phone.

Hit the tuning fork and aim it to the middle of the child's face. Ask the child to turn his head without touching the tuning fork and listen to the sound.

If using a cell phone, pick up the phone and tell the child that someone (a grandparent or friend) is on the phone and wants to say something. Do not let the child grab the phone. Aim it at the middle of the child's body so he will turn his head to listen.

If this does not work, walk into a different room with the child and close the door. Say you think someone is calling his name. Tell him to put his ear up against the door and listen. Hold the door, so the child doesn't choose to open it instead.

Do the exercise three times but not in a row and note which ear the child uses.

Exercise 1. L _____ R _____
Exercise 2. L _____ R _____
Exercise 3. L _____ R _____

▶ *Dominance Profile*

Use this area to log your discovery. If the child used the right in some tasks and the left for others for the same body part, there is no dominance. Check off "Mixed" for ambidextrous.

Hand	Left _____	Right _____	Mixed _____
Foot	Left _____	Right _____	Mixed _____
Eye	Left _____	Right _____	Mixed _____
Ear	Left _____	Right _____	Mixed _____

PRIMITIVE REFLEXES

Primitive reflexes are the basic necessities of survival that are housed in the central nervous system. The development of the central nervous system begins at conception and develops in a regular sequence. Parts of this sequence are identified by the movement patterns that occur at each stage. These are called reflexes. Each reflex plays a part in the necessary growth of the fetus and infant. Each reflex also prepares the way for the next stage of development.

These primitive reflexes should disappear by the age of one. If they don't, it indicates a developmental delay. I have found that as you balance the brain, these primitive reflexes will naturally disappear. If your child seems to get "stuck" or does not improve while doing the At-Home Brain Balance Program, you should have your child professionally evaluated. A trained professional can devise a specific exercise program to correct the problem. This is also true for mixed dominance.

POSTURAL ASSESSMENT

▶ *Head Tilt*

Here you are going to determine if the head tilts right or left. Ask your child to sit straight but don't ask him to hold his head straight. The side of the tilt is usually the side of the weaker hemisphere.

Have your child sit facing you, preferably at eye level. You want him to sit straight and remain still; however, he needs to be in a natural position so he feels comfortable.

Check for a head tilt by observing the bottom of the ear. Record which side is lower.

R_____ L_____

▶ *Eye Balance*

Here you are going to assess for an eye imbalance. Gently position the child's head so that it is level or straight. The head is level when the bottoms of the ears are level facing you.

This will bring out any imbalances in their eyes more.

Ask the child to look straight ahead, either at you or the wall behind you. Look at your child's eyes and observe if one is wider than the other. To detect this, look at the distance between the iris (the colored part of the eye) of each eye and the lower eyelid. Record the eye with the larger distance.

The eye that seems to be larger will usually be on the side of the weak hemisphere.

R_____ L_____

▶ *Fixation*

Some children with right hemisphere deficits are not able to fix their eyes on an object without blinking or moving their eyes for more than 3 seconds. The ability for a child to hold his eyes still and focus on an object or a person is known as fixation. It is very important and is almost always lacking in a child with a right hemisphere weakness.

Point to an object or pick up an object and position it no closer than 18 inches in front of the child's face. Ask the child to stare at the object. Count to three.

Indicate below if the child was able to fixate.

Fixation No _____ Yes _____

▶ *Pupils*

Now you are going to check your child's pupils. You do not want your child to be focusing on something close when you do this. Have the child focus on a spot on the wall behind you, so it is easier to keep the eyes still. Look to see if one of their pupils is larger than the other. You may have to look back and forth several times to see any difference. The larger pupil is usually seen on the side of hemispheric weakness.

Larger Pupil R _____ L _____

▶ *Facial Muscles*

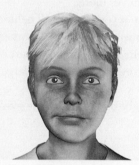

Here you will be checking for facial muscle weakness. The best way to do this is to look at the nasolabial folds. These are the faint lines (in children) that go from the bottom of the nose to the corner of the mouth, as seen in the illustration (in adults these are often called "laugh lines"). When you look closely, these two lines should be equally visible or absent in a child. You may see that one of the creases looks deeper than the other. If there is a noticeable crease, the side where there is no crease or a more shallow crease is usually the side of the weak hemisphere.

If you cannot find the fold, do this: Look at the child's closed mouth when she is neither smiling nor frowning. You may see that one side is slightly lower than the other. Note the side. This and the fainter or absent crease indicate a hemispheric weakness on the same side.

R _____ L _____

▶ *Soft Palate*

You will need a penlight or a flashlight for this assessment. Actually, most children are good at this as long as you don't use a tongue depressor. If the child's tongue gets in the way, use a Q-tip to hold down the front of the tongue. Don't put it toward the back or it will make the child gag.

Have the child open her mouth and say "Ahhhhh." Tilt her head back slightly or crouch down, so you can get a look at the soft palette, or the back roof of the mouth. Have her continue to say "Ahh." Observe the little white stripe that goes from the front to the back of the soft palate that divides it in two. As the child says "Ahh," you will see that the soft palette goes up as the muscles contract. Both sides of the soft palate should go up at the same speed and same distance. You are checking to see if the white stripe in the middle is drawn more to one side or the other. The side that the white stripe moves toward is usually away from the side of the brain that is weak. Record the side that the stripe is moving away from.

R _____ L _____

▶ *Tongue Deviation*

Ask the child to open her mouth slightly and stick out her tongue as far as possible. Look to see if the tongue points to the right or the left. Opposite of what is seen with the soft palette, the tongue will usually point toward the weak hemisphere. Record the side that the tongue is moving toward.

R _____ L _____

▶ *Standing Body Tilt*

You want to be able to see the child's body in this assessment, so have her wear shorts and a T-top (or no top).

Have the child stand straight in front of you. Bend or sit to observe the child at shoulder height. Note if one shoulder is lower than the other. You can also observe this by looking at the child from the back. Note the side of the shoulder tilt. This usually indicates the side of weakness.

A shoulder tilt can also indicate scoliosis (curvature of the spine), so you should have this checked by your child's pediatrician or chiropractor.

R _____ L _____

▶ Elbow Bend

Ask the child to stand up straight in a relaxed natural position, with his arms at his sides. Check for a bend in the elbow and note which elbow is bent more. The side with the more pronounced bend will usually be on the side of hemispheric weakness.

R _____ L _____

▶ Hand Placement

Ask the child to stand up straight in a relaxed natural position, with his arms at his sides and hands relaxed. The thumbs will naturally face forward toward you. You should not see the back of either hand facing you. If they do, this indicates that the arm is rotated in toward the body on that side, signaling an imbalance between the muscles in the front and back of the arm. This is usually seen with a brain imbalance. Check to see if you can see the back of one hand more than the other. Note the side. This is usually on the side of hemispheric weakness.

R _____ L _____

▶ Thumb Strength

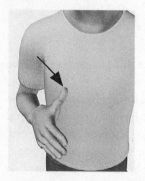

You can do this one thumb at a time, though doing both together will give you a better comparison.

Ask the child to stand up straight in a relaxed natural position. Ask him to make a fist with both hands and stick the thumbs up in the air as straight as possible. Place your thumbs on top of his thumbs, instructing that he not let you push his thumbs down. Gently increase pressure on his thumbs until the muscle fails. Take note if one thumb is weaker than the other. The side of the weaker thumb is usually on the side of the weaker hemisphere.

R _____ L _____

If this didn't work, you can try this instead. You may want to repeat this a few times to get an accurate gauge.

Ask the child to bring the thumb and pinky finger of one hand together on the same hand and hold the position tightly. Say you are going to try to pull the fingers apart but you want him to resist. Gently try to pull the fingers apart until they separate. Do the same with the other hand. The side on which the fingers are the strongest is usually opposite the side of hemispheric weakness.

R _____ L _____

▶ *Big Toe*

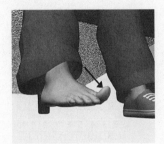

Have the child sit in a chair barefooted and raise one leg straight out. Ask the child to move the big toe in toward her body as far as possible. Tell her to resist as you gently try to push the toe down toward you. Repeat with the other leg and toe. Record the side with the weaker toe. This is the side of hemisphere weakness.

R _____ L _____

▶ *Postural Assessment Results*

Transfer the postural assessment results here. You should see that most, if not all, are either left or right. This correlates to a brain deficiency of the same side.

Head tilt	L _____	R _____
Eye balance	L _____	R _____
Fixation	L _____	R _____
Pupils	L _____	R _____
Facial muscles	L _____	R _____
Soft palate	L _____	R _____
Tongue deviation	L _____	R _____
Standing body tilt	L _____	R _____

Elbow bend	L _____	R _____
Hand placement	L _____	R _____
Thumb strength	L _____	R _____
Big toe	L _____	R _____
TOTAL	L _____	R _____

VESTIBULAR FUNCTION CHECKLIST

The vestibular system is all about balance and spatial awareness. These are signs of a problem in this area. Read each of the following symptoms and place a check in the box that most closely describes your child. A 1 indicates "doesn't apply at all," and a 10 is "almost always." Add up the numbers and record the total. (The lowest possible score is 10, and the highest is 100.)

Exhibits poor balance
1 2 3 4 5 6 7 8 9 10 ☐☐☐☐☐☐☐☐☐☐

Had delayed crawling, standing and/or walking
1 2 3 4 5 6 7 8 9 10 ☐☐☐☐☐☐☐☐☐☐

Poor muscle tone (extremely flexible)
1 2 3 4 5 6 7 8 9 10 ☐☐☐☐☐☐☐☐☐☐

Experiences motion sickness
1 2 3 4 5 6 7 8 9 10 ☐☐☐☐☐☐☐☐☐☐

Dislikes heights, swings, carousels, escalators, elevators
1 2 3 4 5 6 7 8 9 10 ☐☐☐☐☐☐☐☐☐☐

Easily disoriented and/or a poor sense of direction
1 2 3 4 5 6 7 8 9 10 ☐☐☐☐☐☐☐☐☐☐

Clumsy
1 2 3 4 5 6 7 8 9 10 ☐☐☐☐☐☐☐☐☐☐

Difficulty remaining still; may actively seek movement such as spinning and/or rocking
1 2 3 4 5 6 7 8 9 10 ☐☐☐☐☐☐☐☐☐☐

Difficulties with space perception
1 2 3 4 5 6 7 8 9 10 ☐☐☐☐☐☐☐☐☐☐

Walks or walked on toes
1 2 3 4 5 6 7 8 9 10 ☐☐☐☐☐☐☐☐☐☐

Total _____

VESTIBULAR BALANCE ASSESSMENT

The term *Disconnected Kids* is a direct reference to a malfunction of the vestibular, or inner ear, system. The vestibular system is one of the main systems that helps children orient themselves in the earth's gravitational pull. It helps them maintain proper posture and balance. The inner ear balance system, along with the proprioceptive (spatial awareness) system and the oculomotor (eye muscles) system, make up the majority of all stimulus to the brain. The vestibular system works closely with the visual and auditory systems to help with spatial awareness and movement.

A child who has an underactive vestibular system will be kind of clumsy and may never seem to get dizzy when spinning. A child with an overactive vestibular system gets dizzy easily. This is the child who gets motion sickness in the car.

What you will be looking for in this assessment is balance between the right and the left vestibular system. Balance is critical in the vestibular system. If one side is overactive, it will make the other side underactive.

The vestibular system on one side sends its signals to the opposite side of the brain. When a child turns in one direction, it activates the vestibular system on the same side. So if a child spins to the right (clockwise), it turns on the vestibular system in the right ear, and vice versa. This is what you are going to do in these tests. It is called post-rotational nystagmus and it is the best way to assess balance of the vestibular system. Nystagmus is the term used to describe quick involuntary movements of the eyes that occur when the body spins or the head moves quickly. This is what gives us the sensation of vertigo or that the earth is spinning, even if we are still.

The primary vestibular area in the brain that processes vestibular information resides in the right side of the brain and lies very close to the part of the brain that controls the digestive system and the sense of taste or smell, the right frontal insula cortex. This is why you feel nauseous when you are dizzy.

These tests will help determine if your child has a weakness of the right or the left vestibular system. The weak hemisphere will be opposite the weak side of the vestibular system.

For all these tests, you will need a chair with arms that spins easily. The arms are important for the safety of the child so make sure that you only use a chair with arms.

▶ *Post-Rotational (Nystagmus) Tests*

Slow Spin

Have the child sit straight in the chair with the head bent slightly forward and in the middle. Legs must be off the floor and on the chair, either tucked in or Indian style. Instruct the child to keep the head still during the exercise. Start spinning the chair slowly to make sure the child can tolerate the test. You only need to do this for a few seconds. Ask the child to close his eyes and very slowly spin the chair in one direction. It should take 60 seconds to do one full rotation. While you are spinning, instruct the child to point a finger in the direction he is spinning. Also, tell him to let you know when you've stopped spinning the chair. Slowly bring the chair to a stop. Ask the child if he is still spinning. If he says yes, then ask him to tell you when he stops. Once the child says the spinning stopped, have him open his eyes. Ask if he feels dizzy or sick. Then repeat the same exercise in the opposite direction. Note if the child could correctly identify the direction of the motion, when he said the chair stopped spinning, and if he felt dizzy when he opened his eyes. Record the results of both scores.

LEFT SPIN

Direction of spin	L _____	R _____
Accurate stopping	Yes _____	No _____
Dizziness	Yes _____	No _____

RIGHT SPIN

Direction of spin	L _____	R _____
Accurate stopping	Yes _____	No _____
Dizziness	Yes _____	No _____

Fast Spin

If the child can tolerate slow spinning, you are going to speed it up to make the child get dizzy.

Start from the same position as above. With the child's eyes open, spin the chair in one direction ten times. Each full rotation should take 2 seconds. After the tenth rotation stop the child so she is facing you. Tell the child not to look directly at you but up toward the ceiling. You may want to gently grab her head so she doesn't move it around. Quickly check the child's eyes. Both eyes should be moving quickly back and forth. Count how long this continues. Note it in the space below.

When the eyes stop moving, the child should stop feeling dizzy. Make sure the eyes have stopped moving and there is no dizziness before repeating in the other direction. If the eyes are not moving after they stop, this shows a very underactive vestibular system.

Normal eye movement after spinning is 12 to 14 seconds. Less than 12 seconds is considered underactive. Longer than 14 seconds is considered overactive. The underactive side indicates the underactive hemisphere.

Right spin (clockwise) _____ seconds
Left spin (counterclockwise) _____ seconds

Level 1

Feels dizzy after slow spin or can't accurately tell direction of slow spin. No movement of eyes at all after fast spin.

Level 2

Movement of eyes for less than 6 seconds after fast spin.

Level 3

Movement of the eyes for 12 to 14 seconds.

▶ *Vestibular Ocular Reflex*

When we walk, the head bobs up and down in a kind of figure 8 movement. If the eyes moved with the head, the world would be blurry. So we have a reflex that keeps the eyes still and level to the horizon when we walk, run, or move our head. This reflex is called the vestibular ocular reflex.

When the head moves in one direction, the vestibular system signals the eyes to move in the opposite direction at the exact same speed the head is moving. This keeps the eyes still even though the head is moving. If there is an imbalance in the vestibular system, the cerebellum, or the neck and postural muscles, it can affect how well this all works.

A sensitivity on one side means there will be undersensitivity on the other. The undersensitive side can make a child clumsy and bang into things. If overactive, the child will get dizzy and may get motion sick. Here is how you are going to test this reflex.

Have the child sit opposite you in a stationary chair. Hold up your index finger about 18 inches from the front of her nose. Have the child focus both eyes on your finger and tell her to slowly turn her head to one side only as far and as fast as she can while she can still see your finger, then ask her to turn her head back to the middle and stop. Do this ten times to the same side without stopping. The child should be able to keep her eyes fixed on your finger the whole time. If her eyes turn away toward her head motion, this is abnormal. Count how many times the eyes turned away from your finger and toward the direction of the head movement.

The more the eye turns away from the finger, the more the reflex is underactive. If the child is able to maintain contact with the finger but gets dizzy afterward, it is a sign that the reflex is overactive on that side. The underactive reflex will be on the opposite side of the underactive hemisphere. If it is underactive and overactive on both sides equally, this is rare but it is a sign of a general vestibular dysfunction.

LEVEL 1
Eye turns 6 to 10 times.

LEVEL 2
Eye turns 1 to 5 times.

LEVEL 3
No eye turns and no dizziness.

UNDERACTIVITY
R (L hemisphere) _____ L (R hemisphere) _____ Equal _____

▶ *Vestibular Balance Results*

Record the results of the tests here. If the results favor one side, there is weakness in the opposite hemisphere.

Slow Spin (clockwise)	R _____	L _____
Slow Spin (counterclockwise)	R _____	L _____
Fast Spin (clockwise)	R _____	L _____
Fast Spin (counterclockwise)	R _____	L _____
Vestibular ocular reflex	R _____	L _____
TOTAL	R _____	L _____

AUDITORY FUNCTION CHECKLIST

These are the symptoms of a problem with the auditory sensory system. Read each of the following symptoms and place a check in the box that most closely describes your child. A 1 indicates "doesn't apply at all," and a 10 is "almost always." Add up the numbers and record the total. (The lowest possible score is 10 and the highest is 100.)

Concern about hearing as an infant
1 2 3 4 5 6 7 8 9 10
☐ ☐ ☐ ☐ ☐ ☐ ☐ ☐ ☐ ☐

Inability to sing in tune
1 2 3 4 5 6 7 8 9 10
☐ ☐ ☐ ☐ ☐ ☐ ☐ ☐ ☐ ☐

Hypersensitive to sounds
1 2 3 4 5 6 7 8 9 10
☐ ☐ ☐ ☐ ☐ ☐ ☐ ☐ ☐ ☐

Misinterprets questions
1 2 3 4 5 6 7 8 9 10
☐ ☐ ☐ ☐ ☐ ☐ ☐ ☐ ☐ ☐

Confuses similar-sounding words; frequently needs to have words repeated
1 2 3 4 5 6 7 8 9 10
☐ ☐ ☐ ☐ ☐ ☐ ☐ ☐ ☐ ☐

Inability to follow sequential instructions
1 2 3 4 5 6 7 8 9 10
☐ ☐ ☐ ☐ ☐ ☐ ☐ ☐ ☐ ☐

Flat and monotonous voice
1 2 3 4 5 6 7 8 9 10
☐ ☐ ☐ ☐ ☐ ☐ ☐ ☐ ☐ ☐

Hesitant speech
1 2 3 4 5 6 7 8 9 10
☐ ☐ ☐ ☐ ☐ ☐ ☐ ☐ ☐ ☐

Small vocabulary
1 2 3 4 5 6 7 8 9 10
☐ ☐ ☐ ☐ ☐ ☐ ☐ ☐ ☐ ☐

Confusion or reversal of letters
1 2 3 4 5 6 7 8 9 10
☐ ☐ ☐ ☐ ☐ ☐ ☐ ☐ ☐ ☐

Total _____

AUDITORY ASSESSMENT

Many of the children we work with in our clinics have some type of auditory problem. Almost all have hearing that tests normal, yet they don't seem to react to sound in a normal way. Some are undersensitive to sound. In fact, many parents tell me that they thought their child was deaf as an infant.

Many parents of children diagnosed with attention and reading problems have also been diagnosed with some type of auditory processing problem, also referred to as central auditory processing disorder.

What most people are unaware of is that auditory processing, like most sensory detection and processing, is different in the right and the left hemispheres. It is not enough to say the child has a hearing or auditory processing deficit. It must also be determined if it is a *right or left deficiency*. This is important because the problems associated with such a disorder show up differently, and they require different approaches. No sensory function works in isolation. All the senses are dependent on other sensory functions, which are dependent on a baseline level of brain activity.

Most people assume that if a child doesn't respond well to sound, or if he doesn't process sound properly, there must be something wrong with his ears or with his hearing mechanism. In most instances that we see, this is not the case. The hearing pathway and the ears are perfectly normal; the brain is not responding to the sound because brain activity is under threshold. If brain activity is not pulsing at the right speed, it can't keep up with the input of sound. It does not reach a conscious level of awareness.

The baseline level of brain activity comes mainly from the constant flow of input from gravity—that is, input from postural muscles and other tendon, joint, and skin receptors. This is why auditory stimulation alone is not enough to make the brain work as a whole. The big muscles must be worked as well.

The best way to test hearing and auditory processing is through formal testing with an audiologist. If your child has had a hearing test, find out if there was a hearing difference in the two ears. If one ear is hearing less, even if both ears are within normal limits, this may signify an imbalance in the brain. The audiologist, however, may not look at this.

There are simple tests you can perform to see if your child has decreased or unbalanced hearing and processing. Of course, before doing these tests, make sure your child does not have an ear infection, or fluid or wax in his ears at the time of the testing. Get your child's ears checked and have a formal hearing test performed as well.

▶ Tuning Fork Test

You will be using a tuning fork for this assessment. Demonstrate what you are going to do on yourself several times, so you are familiar with the procedure. Also, tell the child exactly what you are going to do and what you want him to do during the process. Quick movements often make a child jump, so you'll actually want to demonstrate without sounding the tuning fork. You want the child to sit still and not move his head or try to grab the instrument.

Explain that you will be hitting the fork and it will make a *ping* sound followed by a low steady *hmmmmmm* sound. Tell the child to let you know when he doesn't hear the sound anymore. Now, hit the tuning fork and put it about 2 to 3 inches from the right (or left) ear. Use a stop watch or count in your head the number of seconds that go by before you get the signal that the sound has stopped. Record the elapsed time. Do this at least two or three times to be certain the results are accurate. The elapsed time should be the same for both ears. Also ask the child if it sounded louder in one ear or the other.

Typically, the sound should be audible for around 60 seconds, depending how hard you hit the tuning fork. Less than 60 seconds indicates reduced sensitivity to sound, either because of poor attention or reduced processing of sound in the brain. This is usually opposite the side of hemispheric weakness. So, note in the space below the side of the brain *opposite* the reduced hearing.

Another way you can do this exercise is with vibration. This will make your results even more accurate.

As you strike the tuning fork, you will feel the vibration in your fingers. As you count, take note how many seconds after the vibration stops that the child stops hearing the sound. The child should hear the sound for 10 to 20 seconds after you stop feeling the vibration in your fingers. It should be equally as long on both sides.

Side *opposite* weak hearing ear   R _____   L _____

▶ *Simultaneous Sound (Dichotic Listening) Test*

This test should be done with the eyes closed. If the child is too distracted to do this, you will need to cover her eyes so she can concentrate on what she is hearing. Again, this test may take some practice, so try it on yourself or your spouse first to make sure you are doing it correctly. The idea of this test is to present the exact same sound to both ears at the exact same time. You will be checking to see if the child hears the sound first in one ear before the other. You want to be eye level, so you should kneel in front of the child or have the child stand on a steady chair.

Stand or kneel facing the child. Extend your arms so your hands are 18 inches from both of your child's ears. Rub your thumbs against your fingers and ask if the child can hear the sound. If not, slowly move your hands closer to the ears at the same speed and distance, and ask the child to signal you when she hears the sound. Ask if she heard it in both ears or just one ear. If it is just one ear, continue to get closer until she hears the sound. Sound heard first in only one ear indicates a weakness on the opposite side of the brain of the ear that was slower in hearing. Note the sound opposite from where the sound was first detected. Note the side of decreased hearing.

Sound in both ears at the same time _____

or

Side opposite the ear where the sound
was detected L _____   R _____

LEVEL 1

Child hears sound for less than 30 seconds in either or both ears or has a significant or large difference between the two ears on either test.

LEVEL 2

Child hears sound for less than 45 seconds in either or both ears or has a moderate difference between the two ears on either test.

LEVEL 3

Child hears the sound for 60 seconds in both ears and has no difference between the two ears.

▶ *Auditory Dysfunction Results*

Transfer the results here.

Tuning Fork Test	R _____	L _____	
Simultaneous Sound Test	R _____	L _____	No Difference _____
TOTAL	R _____	L _____	No Difference _____

•   •   •

VISUAL DYSFUNCTION CHECKLIST

This checklist focuses on symptoms that make reading difficult. If you are not sure, talk to your child's teacher or go through some reading exercises with your child. Read each of the following symptoms and place a check in the box that most closely describes your child. A 1 indicates "doesn't apply at all," and a 10 is "almost always." Add up the numbers and record the total. (The lowest possible score is 10 and the highest is 100.)

	1 2 3 4 5 6 7 8 9 10
Misreads words	□ □ □ □ □ □ □ □ □ □
Misses or repeats words or lines	□ □ □ □ □ □ □ □ □ □
Reads slowly	□ □ □ □ □ □ □ □ □ □
Needs to use finger or marker as a pointer	□ □ □ □ □ □ □ □ □ □
Inability to remember what was read	□ □ □ □ □ □ □ □ □ □
Poor concentration	□ □ □ □ □ □ □ □ □ □
Poor focus while reading, i.e., letters move or jump around on the page	□ □ □ □ □ □ □ □ □ □
Crooked or sloped handwriting	□ □ □ □ □ □ □ □ □ □
Letters appear out of balance with one eye covered or while trying to read sideways	□ □ □ □ □ □ □ □ □ □
Sensitivity to light	□ □ □ □ □ □ □ □ □ □

Total _____

VISUAL ASSESSMENT

Vision is the most complex sense to test, for several reasons:

■ It is the only sense that is directly dependent on the movement of muscles.

- Eyes have to detect both light and movement.
- Sometimes eyes must move in perfect concert, as in tracking something slowly or reading a book, but they sometimes must move in the opposite direction, such as when looking at a schoolbook and watching the blackboard.
- Some eye movements are voluntary but most movements are involuntary.
- The muscles of the pupils of the eyes need to contract and relax smoothly to help focus close and far away.

On page 35, I described that there are two different visual systems—the where and the what. The where system is not sensitive to color, sees things faster, and is more interested in the big picture. It's the right brain system. The what system is very sensitive to color, sees things more slowly, and focuses on details. It is the left brain system.

The muscles of the eye are also proprioceptive, meaning they help us feel ourselves in space. Studies show that if we place very small vibrators around the eyes, we can alter individuals' perceptions of their bodies in space or make them feel as if they are moving in a particular direction. This tricks the brain into thinking the body is moving. This illustrates that the eye muscles are powerful messengers and can even override what the person is actually seeing.

All of these factors are separate from 20/20 vision. People think that 20/20 vision is all that matters, but in fact, it is probably the least important function of the eye and the visual system. Some children are born with a weak eye muscle. Their eye may be turned in or out on one side. This is called strabismus. We have all had the experience of talking to someone whose one eye is focused on you but the other eye is somewhat "off." Though this has traditionally been looked at as an eye problem, we can now see that the issue may have more to do with the brain.

For proper vision, both eyes must work in perfect concert. When one eye is weak or "lazy," it means a child can only see with one eye at a time. Obviously, this interferes with good vision. Only the child does not recognize this. Each eye can see when the other is shut, but when both eyes are open, the brain ignores the images in the one eye and only sees out of the good eye. At one time, doctors believed this was caused by a weak eye, but we now know that it is caused by the brain being out of rhythm.

Vision comes from the occipital lobe. The right lobe gets vision from the left half of both eyes and the left lobe gets vision from the right half of both eyes. If one eye is blind, the occipital lobe will take over both sides. If the two hemispheres of the brain are not in sync, however, the occipital lobes are desynchronized. The brain gets two completely different visions of the world. The brain can't fuse the images together, but instead of seeing double, it ignores the bad eye and focuses only on what it sees out of the good eye.

When the problem is slight, vision can adjust and compensate. However, the worse the problem, the worse the symptoms will be.

▶ *Light Sensitivity Test*

Using a penlight or small flashlight on the lowest setting, focus the beam in the outside corner of one eye. Count how long it takes for the pupil to constrict and enlarge completely back to its original size. Depending on how bright the light is, the pupils should normally stay constricted for about 10 seconds. If the pupil constricts quickly and dilates right away, this usually shows a weakness in the brain on the opposite side. Note the time. Repeat on the other side. Also note if the child's eyes tear or if they are so hypersensitive to the light that you can't perform the exercise. The weak hemisphere is usually opposite the eye that dilates first.

Right eye _____ seconds
Tearing   Y _____ N _____
Sensitivity   Y _____ N _____
Left eye _____ seconds
Tearing   Y _____ N _____
Sensitivity   Y _____ N _____

LEVEL 1
The child turns away from the light or closes her eyes.

LEVEL 2
The child's eye constricts then dilates quickly. It takes less than 10 seconds to dilate.

LEVEL 3

The child's pupil constricts and then returns to fully dilated in 10 to 15 seconds.

▶ *Fast Tracking (Saccades) Test*

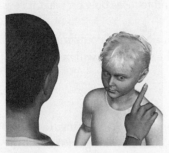

Fast tracking is a very important vision function. It is critical in reading, for example, when the eye jumps from one line to the next. Many children with FDS have great difficulty doing this and may overshoot or undershoot the target. This makes reading difficult and very slow.

This testing will allow you to determine which side of the brain is underactive, slower, and underconnected.

Sit directly in front of your child at eye level. The child should sit tall with the head straight. If you detect a head tilt, try to gently straighten the head. Hold your pointer fingers about 12 inches from your child's face and about 30 degrees out to the side, as illustrated. Tell the child to stare at your face. Say that you are going to wiggle your finger and tell the child to turn her eyes to the finger without moving her head as soon as she detects it. Her eyes should move quickly to your finger in one smooth movement. Watch her eyes carefully to see if she overshoots when she turns to focus on your finger. You will know this because she will move the eyes again back to the finger if she went too far. Look for that second movement back to the finger. When you say okay, the child should turn her eyes back and stare at your nose. Repeat by wiggling your fingers in a random pattern so the child cannot predict where you start or stop. Do this a total of five times. Repeat on the other side. The side of the brain opposite the direction of the eyes that overshoots will be the side of the weak hemisphere.

Side opposite the overshoot   R _____ L _____

LEVEL 1

The child cannot do the activity or she overshoots every time in either direction, or she has a significant difference between the speed of movement of both eyes.

LEVEL 2

The child overshoots two times in either direction or she has a significant difference between the speed of movement of both eyes.

LEVEL 3

There is no overshooting, and speed of movement is equal on both sides.

▶ *Slow Tracking (Pursuit) Test*

Only humans and the highest level of primates can perform conscious voluntary slow tracking movements with the eyes. Obviously, this means that this has something to do with having a more sophisticated brain. Therefore, measuring this ability in children is very important. If a child can perform smooth, slow tracking movements while following a target both left and right, it is a good sign of brain development. This is also very easy to assess.

The child's head needs to remain still during the exercise. If the head moves, put your hand on top of the head to hold it in place.

Have the child seated in front of you so that you are face-to-face. Tell the child to sit straight with the head level and still. Place your index finger at eye level and to the left of the child's head. Tell the child to turn her eyes and follow your finger as you move it slowly to the right and as far as the eyes can follow. It should take about 6 seconds to get from one side to the next. Reverse the direction. If the child has trouble, or if the eyes are moving more slowly or if they are jumping back and forth more following your finger to one side, it is a sign of a hemispheric deficiency in the same side. If she cannot follow your finger in either direction, it shows poor fixation ability, which is a right hemisphere weakness.

R _____ L _____ No fixation _____

LEVEL 1

The child cannot follow the finger or has significant jumping of eyes or slowness in either direction or has a significant imbalance in speed and accuracy of tracking between the two sides.

LEVEL 2

The child can follow the finger but has significant jumping of eyes in either direction or has a significant imbalance in speed and accuracy of tracking between the two sides.

LEVEL 3

The child can track the finger smoothly to both sides with no jumping and no difference in speed in either direction.

▶ *Crossing Eyes (Convergence/Divergence) Test*

The ability to bring both eyes toward the nose at the same time, or crossing the eyes, is known as convergence. This is another skill that we assume children can do but it is no guarantee. Between 30 and 50 percent of all children diagnosed with ADHD cannot cross their eyes. I have found this is also true with most children with a right hemisphere weakness.

If the child cannot cross his eyes smoothly, it affects close-range reading. It also makes it difficult to copy from a blackboard. If the eyes can't work together, then it is likely that the two hemispheres are not working together as well.

Have the child sit straight with the head straight. Face the child at eye level. Raise your index finger about 18 inches in front of his nose. Tell him to follow your finger with both eyes as you slowly move it in toward his nose. Ask him how many fingers he sees. If the answer is two fingers, it is an indication that the eyes are not aligned and they may have a more severe muscle weakness. You should be able to get 1 to 2 inches in front of the nose before he sees two fingers. Move your finger back till he says he sees only one finger. Check the child's eyes to see if one is turned out. The eye that is turned out is the weak eye and usually indicates a hemispheric weakness on the same side. If he cannot cross his eyes at all, it shows a right hemisphere weakness. If the child can successfully do the exercise, repeat it five to ten times and observe if one eye fatigues and turns out. If one tires and turns out early, it can also indicate a brain weakness on the same side. Record the results below.

R_____ L_____ Cannot cross eyes _____

. . .

LEVEL 1
Cannot cross eyes closer than 12 inches from nose without seeing double.

LEVEL 2
Cannot cross eyes closer than 6 inches from nose without seeing double.

LEVEL 3
Can cross eyes equally up to 2 inches from nose without seeing double.

▶ *Vision Assessment Results*

Transfer the vision assessment results here. If the results weigh heavily to one side, it indicates an imbalance on that side of the brain.

Light Sensitivity Test	R _____	L _____
Fast Track Test	R _____	L _____
Slow Track Test	R _____	L _____
Cross Eyes Test	R _____	L _____
TOTAL	R _____	L _____

PROPRIOCEPTIVE FUNCTION CHECKLIST

This checklist will help judge how well your child feels his or her body in space. Read each of the following symptoms and place a check in the box that most closely describes your child. A 1 indicates "doesn't apply at all," and a 10 is "almost always." Add up the numbers and record the total. (The lowest possible score is 10 and the highest is 100.)

Poor posture

1 2 3 4 5 6 7 8 9 10
☐ ☐ ☐ ☐ ☐ ☐ ☐ ☐ ☐ ☐

Constant fidgeting or moving

1 2 3 4 5 6 7 8 9 10
☐ ☐ ☐ ☐ ☐ ☐ ☐ ☐ ☐ ☐

Excessive desire to be held

1 2 3 4 5 6 7 8 9 10
☐ ☐ ☐ ☐ ☐ ☐ ☐ ☐ ☐ ☐

Provokes fights

1 2 3 4 5 6 7 8 9 10
☐ ☐ ☐ ☐ ☐ ☐ ☐ ☐ ☐ ☐

	1	2	3	4	5	6	7	8	9	10
Hooks feet around legs of desk for support	☐	☐	☐	☐	☐	☐	☐	☐	☐	☐
Problem identifying body parts in space	☐	☐	☐	☐	☐	☐	☐	☐	☐	☐
Bumps into things often	☐	☐	☐	☐	☐	☐	☐	☐	☐	☐
Poor balance	☐	☐	☐	☐	☐	☐	☐	☐	☐	☐
Rocks body or bangs head	☐	☐	☐	☐	☐	☐	☐	☐	☐	☐
Does not like heights	☐	☐	☐	☐	☐	☐	☐	☐	☐	☐

Total _____

PROPRIOCEPTIVE ASSESSMENT

Proprioception is the ability to know where one's body is in space relative to gravity and where it is relative to itself and other people or objects. I consider the proprioceptive system the most important influence on other sensory systems and the brain as a whole. Other doctors believe the vestibular system is more important, but I disagree. Research has proven that a person can compensate fairly well for a vestibular loss but can never compensate for a severe proprioceptive loss.

The funny thing about the proprioceptive sense is that when it is diminished or lost, no one—parents or child—realizes it because it is the one sense that is mostly subconscious. We are much more familiar and consciously aware of the other senses such as vision, hearing, smell, taste, and touch. Proprioception, however, is more essential to the brain because it is the only sense that is constant. It works closely with the vestibular system, which also is mostly subconscious.

When children first start to move and walk, they have to actively think about their movements. This makes it hard for the brain to concentrate and learn anything else. If a child doesn't get it—if he is clumsy and walks oddly—it is hard for him to move on to other skills because his brain is so preoccupied with trying to control movements. When a child learns to walk and move naturally, however, the brain no longer has to think about these things. Movement becomes subconscious.

Muscle tone is also a good indicator of proprioception. If the child has low muscle tone, then the muscles and tendons and joints will be undersensitive to movement because the body has to move a lot more before the brain reacts to that movement. This is what makes movements appear clumsy, slow, and uncoordinated.

▶ Standing Balance (Rhomberg) Test

Have your child stand facing you in a relaxed position and barefoot. Ask him to move his feet together so the ankles touch. Note if he remains straight or sways to one side or the other. Stand close enough so you can catch him if he falls. If he can stay balanced, ask him to close his eyes. Again, look for a sway. A sway or fall indicates a hemispheric weakness in the opposite direction of the sway. Record the side of the brain that is opposite the sway.

L _____ R _____ No sway _____

▶ One Foot in Front of the Other (Manns) Test

If your child did fine on the previous test, these two tests will be more challenging.

Have the child stand straight, barefoot, and relaxed with feet together. Tell the child to put one foot directly in front of the other. Note if he sways to one side. Be close to catch him in case he falls. As he keeps the pose, ask him to close his eyes. A sway to one side indicates a hemispheric weakness on the opposite side of the sway. Record the side opposite the sway.

Eyes open   L _____ R _____
Eyes closed   L _____ R _____

▶ One Leg Stand

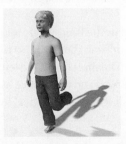

Have the child stand barefoot in front of you. Ask him to lift one leg bent at the knee. Use a stop watch or count silently the seconds the child can remain upright without swaying or needing to grab on to something. She should be able to maintain the position for 30 seconds. If successful, ask her to repeat the exercise with eyes closed. She should be able to do this for 10 seconds. Repeat with the opposite leg. Repeat the test three times to verify your counting. A sway or fall on one side indicates a hemispheric deficiency on the opposite side of the sway. The side of the shorter balancing time also indicates a deficiency on the opposite side of the brain. Record the side opposite the sway.

Longer balancing time: L _____ R _____
Shorter balancing time: L _____ R _____

LEVEL 1

Stand with one foot in front of the other. Eyes open without falling for 30 seconds.

LEVEL 2

One leg stand with eyes open for 30 seconds without falling or putting foot down.

LEVEL 3

One leg stand with eyes closed for 30 seconds without falling or putting foot down.

▶ Core Stability Test

The core muscles are mainly in the trunk and abdomen. Weakness and poor muscle tone in these muscles are usually due to or can cause poor proprioceptive awareness. Because these muscles are mainly under subconscious control, exercises cannot be done consciously.

The left brain controls most conscious or voluntary movements, especially of small muscles of the hands and feet. Lifting weights, for example, are voluntary muscle movements. The muscles that stabilize the body contract involuntary. This is why conscious exercise won't strengthen these muscles.

The key to stability is a balance of the muscles in the front, back, and sides of the trunk. Normally, the spinal muscles in back should be 30 to 50 percent stronger than the abdominal muscles. The muscles on the left side of the spine should have about the same strength and endurance as the muscles on the right. This balance, plus overall strength, is critical to stability and balance.

A child may appear to have weak leg and arm muscles when, in fact, it is the stabilizing big muscles of the spine that are weak. If the foundation is weak, the arm and leg muscles will appear weak. Sitting inactivates these muscles and will make them weak or lead to delayed development of muscle tone. This is another reason why TV and video games are bad for your child.

▶ Supine Bridge Core Test

LEVEL 1

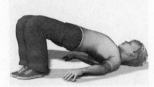

Have the child lie on the floor, hands by the side for stability and legs shoulder-width apart. Ask the child to lift his trunk off the floor so the spine is straight. You can put your hands under his backside to help him lift but don't keep it there. Have him hold this position still for as long as possible. Use a stop watch or count to yourself how long he can hold the position. If he starts to shake, bend, or collapse, encourage him once to keep going, but if he can't correct this, stop counting. A small child should be able to maintain this position for at least 30 seconds; an older child should hold this for 60 seconds.

Time _____

LEVEL 2

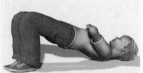

If the child achieved Level 1, give him a 10-second rest and have him do this exercise. It eliminates some of the stability and adds resistance to the muscles, making the exercise harder to do.

While still lying on the floor, have the child put his knees together and cross his arms over his chest. Ask him again to lift his trunk off the floor and hold the same spine-straight position. Count the number of seconds he can hold the position. Record it below. A child who can do Level 2 should be able to hold this position for 60 seconds.

Time _____

LEVEL 3

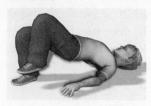

If the child achieves Level 2 without a problem, have him do this exercise. This takes away even more stability and adds more resistance.

Assume the same position as Level 1. Have him lift one leg off the floor about an inch. Count how long he can steadily hold this position and record it below. Switch legs and repeat. A child should be able to hold the position in each leg for 30 seconds. Record it below.

Time _____

▶ *Prone Bridge Core Stability Test*

LEVEL 1

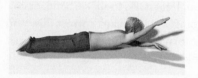

Have the child lie belly down on the floor with arms stretched out next to the head, which should be down and in the middle. Ask the child to raise his head and one arm off the floor, keeping his arm perfectly straight. Ask him to hold this position for as long as possible up to 15 seconds. Stop counting if he drops or bends his arm at all or drops his head. Count how long he can hold this position and record it below. Repeat this with all four limbs separately while lifting the head. Stop counting as soon as any part of the position lets go.

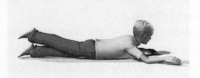

Right arm time _____ seconds
Left arm time _____ seconds
Right leg time _____ seconds
Left leg time _____ seconds

LEVEL 2

If he is able to hold all four limbs separately for 15 seconds, advance to the Level 2 position.

Have the child assume the same position and ask him to lift his head, one arm, and the opposite leg off the floor. Count how long he can keep the position. Relax for 10 seconds.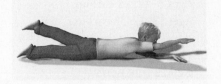
Switch arm and leg and repeat. If he drops arm, head, or leg or bends arm or leg, stop counting. He should be able to do each exercise for 30 seconds on each side. If he fails on either side, he has failed this assessment.

      Right arm and left leg time _____ seconds

      Left arm and right leg time _____ seconds

LEVEL 3

If the child can maintain Level 2 for 30 seconds, have him do this exercise.

Assume the same starting position and ask the child to lift all four limbs off the floor in a Superman position. Ask him to keep the position for as long as possible up to 60 seconds.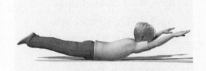

      Time _____ seconds

▶ Curl-Ups

Have the child lie on a flat cushioned and clean surface with knees bent and feet about 12 inches from his backside. Put your hands over his feet for support. Ask him to cross his arms and place his palms on his shoulders. Now ask him to raise his trunk and curl up until his elbows touch his thighs. Ask him to lie back down so the shoulder blades touch the floor, for one curl-up. Continue to do this for 1 minute while counting aloud. The goal is to do as many as possible fluidly without error in 1 minute. He should be able to do the number that matches his age and sex below.

LEVEL 1

GOALS FOR BOYS AND GIRLS
Ages 4–7: 15 curl-ups
Ages 8–12: 25 curl-ups
Ages 13–17: 35 curl-ups

LEVEL 2

GOALS FOR BOYS
Ages 4–7: 25 curl-ups
Ages 8–12: 35 curl-ups
Ages 13–17: 45 curl-ups

GOALS FOR GIRLS
Ages 4–7: 25 curl-ups
Ages 8–12: 35 curl-ups
Ages 13–17: 40 curl-ups

LEVEL 3

GOALS FOR BOYS
Ages 4–7: 35 curl-ups
Ages 8–12: 45 curl-ups
Ages 13–17: 55 curl-ups

GOALS FOR GIRLS
Ages 4–7: 35 curl-ups
Ages 8–12: 45 curl-ups
Ages 13–17: 50 curl-ups

▶ *Right-Angle Push-Ups*

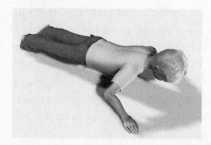

Have the child lie facedown on the floor in the classic push-up position: hands under shoulders, fingers straight, and legs straight, parallel, and slightly apart with the toes supporting the feet. Ask the child to push up, keeping the back and knees straight and then lower the body until there is a 90-degree angle at the elbows. Place your hands on the child's hands so his shoulders touch your hands when he goes back to the floor. The entire exercise should take 3 seconds. Keep track of the number. He should be able to do the number that matches his age and sex below.

LEVEL 1

GOALS FOR BOYS
Ages 4–7: 5 push-ups
Ages 8–12: 10 push-ups
Ages 13–17: 15 push-ups

GOALS FOR GIRLS
Ages 4–7: 5 push-ups
Ages 8–12: 10 push-ups
Ages 13–17: 15 push-ups

LEVEL 2

GOALS FOR BOYS
Ages 4–7: 5 push-ups
Ages 8–12: 15 push-ups
Ages 13–17: 30 push-ups

GOALS FOR GIRLS
Ages 4–7: 5 push-ups
Ages 8–12: 10 push-ups
Ages 13–17: 15 push-ups

LEVEL 3

GOALS FOR BOYS
Ages 4–7: 15 push-ups
Ages 8–12: 25 push-ups
Ages 13–17: 45 push-ups

GOALS FOR GIRLS
Ages 4–7: 15 push-ups
Ages 8–12: 20 push-ups
Ages 13–17: 25 push-ups

▶ *Proprioception Assessment Results*

Record the results of the assessments here. If the results lean heavily to one side, it is an indication of a deficiency in the other side.

Standing Balance Test   R _____ L _____

One Foot in Front of the Other Test   R _____ L _____

One Leg Stand   R _____ L _____

Core Stability Test   R _____ L _____

Supine Bridge Core Test   R _____ L _____

Prone Bridge Core Stability Test

Level 1   R _____ L _____

Level 2   R _____ L _____

Level 3   R _____ L _____

Curl-Ups

Level 1   R _____ L _____

Level 2   R _____ L _____

Level 3   R _____ L _____

Right-Angle Push-Ups

Level 1   R _____ L _____

Level 2   R _____ L _____

Level 3   R _____ L _____

Total   R _____ L _____

TACTILE FUNCTION CHECKLIST

These symptoms indicated either under or oversensitivity to touch. Read each of the following symptoms and place a check in the box that most closely describes your child. A 1 indicates "doesn't apply at all," and a 10 is "almost always." Add up the numbers and record the total. (The lowest possible score is 10, and the highest is 100.)

▶ *Hypotactile (Undersensitivity) Symptoms*

Hypotactile to most things   1 2 3 4 5 6 7 8 9 10
                                        ☐ ☐ ☐ ☐ ☐ ☐ ☐ ☐ ☐ ☐

Doesn't notice or respond when cut
1 2 3 4 5 6 7 8 9 10

High threshold for pain
1 2 3 4 5 6 7 8 9 10

Doesn't sense the feeling of cold or hot
1 2 3 4 5 6 7 8 9 10

Craves contact sports
1 2 3 4 5 6 7 8 9 10

Doesn't notice when sits down on an object
1 2 3 4 5 6 7 8 9 10

Provokes roughhousing or fighting
1 2 3 4 5 6 7 8 9 10

Is not ticklish
1 2 3 4 5 6 7 8 9 10

Compulsively touches
1 2 3 4 5 6 7 8 9 10

Acts like a bull in a china shop
1 2 3 4 5 6 7 8 9 10

▶ Hypertactile (Oversensitivity) Symptoms

Seems hypersensitive all the time
1 2 3 4 5 6 7 8 9 10

Dislikes playing sports
1 2 3 4 5 6 7 8 9 10

Dislikes being touched
1 2 3 4 5 6 7 8 9 10

Hates tags on clothes
1 2 3 4 5 6 7 8 9 10

Has allergic skin reactions
1 2 3 4 5 6 7 8 9 10

Hates makeup and/or jewelry
1 2 3 4 5 6 7 8 9 10

Has poor body temperature control
1 2 3 4 5 6 7 8 9 10

Does not like clothing on arms or legs
1 2 3 4 5 6 7 8 9 10

Has a low external pain threshold
1 2 3 4 5 6 7 8 9 10

Doesn't like touching
1 2 3 4 5 6 7 8 9 10

Total _____

TACTILE ASSESSMENT

Tactile awareness is the ability to feel touch. Many children with FDS have an abnormal sense of touch. More are undersensitive to touch and pain rather than hypersensitive.

The skin contains receptors for both light and deep touch. This, along with the vestibular and proprioceptive senses, is important for the ability to feel oneself in space. If a child does sense touch, it affects her in a number of ways. Tactile awareness, especially of the feet, is very important for balance. It is also important for the child to develop a normal "map" of the body in her brain. Receptors in the left brain regulate the sense of touch on the opposite side of the body. The receptors in the right brain mostly control touch on the left side but also control touch on the right side. This has to do with the right brain's job of seeing the "big picture."

Both undersensitivity and hypersensitivity to touch are signs of underactivity in the brain, especially the right side. Many parents think their child is a little toughy because he didn't cry when he got hurt. However, it is really a sign that the child doesn't have a normal feeling for pain and touch.

Hypersensitivity is also due to underactivity of the brain but it is better than undersensitivity. This is the child that hates to be touched or is hypersensitive to the feeling of tags on shirts or particular types of clothing.

Tactile awareness is important also from a hemispheric perspective. Most often, children are undersensitive to touch but they are much more undersensitive on one side of the body than the other. The undersensitive side of the body is usually opposite the slower, more underactive side of the brain.

▶ *Tactile Sensitivity*

Cover the child's eyes. Using a soft paintbrush, lightly stroke the inside of one forearm and then the other forearm. If you don't have a paintbrush, you can use your fingertips. Ask the child if it felt the same on both arms. If the answer is no, ask on which arm the feeling was the strongest. Repeat three times. Record the arm with the strongest sensation.

L _____ R _____ Both arms the same _____

Repeat the same exercise on the leg above the knee. Repeat three times. Record the leg on which the child felt the strongest sensation.

L _____ R _____ Both legs the same _____

▶ Simultaneous Touch (Extinction) Test

With two brushes or your fingers, gently stroke both forearms at the same time. Make sure you press down equally. As you are stroking, ask him if the feeling is more noticeable on one arm. Repeat three times. Record the side of most intensity. Do the same exercise on the top of the leg. Repeat three times. Record the side of most intensity.

R _____ L _____ Both arms the same _____

▶ Number Tracing (Graphestesia) Test

This test also should be performed with eyes closed. Explain what you will be doing and demonstrate it first so he can watch.

With eyes covered, have the child sit with arms outstretched and palms up. With the eraser end of a pencil, trace a digit from 0 to 9 on one arm and ask him to identify the number. Write the number in the child's style as if he were writing the number so he will recognize it. Do this a total of three times with three different numbers. Repeat on the other side. The side opposite the side of the most inaccuracies indicates the deficient side. Note this side.

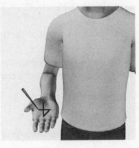

Deficient Side L _____ R _____

Use the symptom checklist to determine the level.

▶ Tactile Assessment Results

Transfer the results here. The side with the most checks indicates a deficiency in the opposite side of the brain.

Tactile Sensitivity R _____ L _____

Simultaneous Touch (Extinction) Test R _____ L _____

Number Tracing (Graphestesia) Test R _____ L _____

Total   R _____ L _____

OLFACTORY FUNCTION CHECKLIST

These two checklists will help you ascertain if your child has a deficiency in the senses of smell and taste. One list checks for oversensitivity and the other undersensitivity. Read each of the symptoms in both lists and place a check in the box that most closely describes your child. A 1 indicates "doesn't apply at all," and a 10 is "almost always." Add up the numbers and record the total. (The lowest possible score is 10, and the highest is 100.) Total each list.

▶ *Hypersensitive Smell and Taste Checklist*

Exhibits increased sensitivity to taste and smell

1	2	3	4	5	6	7	8	9	10
☐	☐	☐	☐	☐	☐	☐	☐	☐	☐

Gags at the smell of certain foods

1	2	3	4	5	6	7	8	9	10
☐	☐	☐	☐	☐	☐	☐	☐	☐	☐

Avoids going to bathroom at the risk of wetting pants because the smell is repugnant

1	2	3	4	5	6	7	8	9	10
☐	☐	☐	☐	☐	☐	☐	☐	☐	☐

Prefers bland foods

1	2	3	4	5	6	7	8	9	10
☐	☐	☐	☐	☐	☐	☐	☐	☐	☐

Avoids children with dirty or smelly clothes

1	2	3	4	5	6	7	8	9	10
☐	☐	☐	☐	☐	☐	☐	☐	☐	☐

Complains about others' bad breath

1	2	3	4	5	6	7	8	9	10
☐	☐	☐	☐	☐	☐	☐	☐	☐	☐

Misbehaves after house is cleaned with solvents

1	2	3	4	5	6	7	8	9	10
☐	☐	☐	☐	☐	☐	☐	☐	☐	☐

Is sensitive to smoke

1	2	3	4	5	6	7	8	9	10
☐	☐	☐	☐	☐	☐	☐	☐	☐	☐

Avoids foods and places with strong cooking smells

1	2	3	4	5	6	7	8	9	10
☐	☐	☐	☐	☐	☐	☐	☐	☐	☐

Sniffs everything

1	2	3	4	5	6	7	8	9	10
☐	☐	☐	☐	☐	☐	☐	☐	☐	☐

▶ *Hyposensitive Smell Checklist*

	1 2 3 4 5 6 7 8 9 10
Never comments on strong smells	☐☐☐☐☐☐☐☐☐☐
Never notices baking smells, such as cookies	☐☐☐☐☐☐☐☐☐☐
Overfills mouth	☐☐☐☐☐☐☐☐☐☐
Avoids foods because of the way it looks	☐☐☐☐☐☐☐☐☐☐
Never sniffs	☐☐☐☐☐☐☐☐☐☐
Hates to eat, even sweets	☐☐☐☐☐☐☐☐☐☐
Chews on objects like pens	☐☐☐☐☐☐☐☐☐☐
Does not notice strong smells like something burning	☐☐☐☐☐☐☐☐☐☐
Eats indiscriminately; will reach for anything, even toxic household products	☐☐☐☐☐☐☐☐☐☐
Is an extremely picky eater	☐☐☐☐☐☐☐☐☐☐

Total _____

OLFACTORY ASSESSMENT

Smell is the sense most people take for granted but it is more important than most parents think.

When our tests confirm that a child has a problematic sense of smell, it often surprises the parents. But the truth is that if your child can't smell, you will almost never realize that on your own. It is hard to tell if a child's sense of smell is diminished or absent, especially if a child never had a good sense of smell to begin with. It is easier to know if your child is hypersensitive to smell, because your child will sniff at and comment on everything.

Most children with FDS have something abnormal with their sense of smell. Ask yourself a few questions. Does your child ever comment on cooking smells, for example? Does he react to strong smells like something burning? Or does your child overreact to smells and complain about them all the time?

Smell and taste are virtually inseparable. Of the two, however, smell is more important. We've all experienced the lack of taste from a snuffy nose cold. Without smell, there is not much interest in taste. Also, without a sense of smell, a child is not able to recognize a smell that signals danger, such as gas.

However, when it comes to the developing brain, a problem with smell is more significant than missing out on the pleasure of food. The sense of smell involves the higher processing centers of the brain, so if this area of the brain is not developing properly, a child most likely will also have trouble with other important facets of life that are controlled in this part of the brain. This can show up as poor emotional awareness, socialization problems, immune and digestive problems, an inability to pay attention, and possibly even impulsive obsessive behaviors. However, when we bring out a child's sense of smell, we see a correction in these troubles as well.

Children with a poor sense of smell are, no surprise, picky eaters. And in most cases, it is because they have a very poor sense of both smell *and* taste. They rely more on how food looks and how it feels in the mouth.

As with the other senses, there is a hemispheric relationship to smell. The right half is more sensitive to bad smells and the left is more sensitive to pleasant smells. I worked with one child with Asperger's who told me he could detect good smells but he didn't recognize bad smells that others in his family could detect.

▶ Sense of Smell Test

When testing your child's sense of smell, you'll want to measure the ability to detect smell in general but also the smell sensitivity in one nostril versus the other. To assess the sense of smell accurately, you will need three things: essential oils, cotton balls, and several empty film canisters. You may already have them in your house. If not, essential oils are available at most health food stores and many department stores. You can get empty film canisters at a photo store. They usually just get thrown out, so they are usually happy to give them away. If you cannot get film canisters, find containers that are small, clean, look the same, and that a child cannot see in. Children are very clever and you want to make sure that they can't identify any canister with a specific aroma. The idea is to put a few drops of the aromatic oil on a cotton ball and deposit it in a canister. Do this with several different aromas. Choose something familiar that your child will recognize such as lemon, orange, apple, strawberry, or peppermint. Instead of essential oils, you can use anything with a strong scent, such as coffee or chocolate. Do not mark the canisters; you want them all to look the same.

Before you do this test, practice it on your child. Make it like a game, so the child gets involved. I always tell children that we are going to do a "smell game." They end up really enjoying it—and you get valuable information. Smell is the only sense that does not cross over to the opposite side of the brain.

Ask the child to close his eyes (or blindfold him, if necessary) and close one nostril with his finger. Hold the canister about 12 inches from his nose. Ask him to breathe in and ask if he smells anything. Start bringing it closer to the nose, inch by inch, and ask him to tell you when he smells something. When he detects the smell, ask him to identify it. Note how far from the nose detection occurred and if the identification was correct. Repeat with the other nostril and tell him the smell may or may not be the same. It is part of the game. A child should be able to detect a strong, familiar smell at a distance of 8 to 10 inches. The side of decreased smell is on the same side as the weak hemisphere.

Smell distance (Detection) R _____ inches L _____ inches

Unable to identify smell (Identification) R _____ L _____

Use the symptom checklist to determine the level.

▶ *Olfactory Assessment Results*

Transfer the results here. The checked side indicates a weakness in the same hemisphere.

Sense of Smell Test R _____ L _____

HEMISPHERIC ASSESSMENT IDENTIFICATION

The assessment tests you just performed should correspond with the results of the Master Hemispheric Checklist in determining the side of the functional weakness. These assessments, however, have now helped you determine the brain function that is causing the imbalance. In the first column of the following table, record whether the assessment indicated a left or a right imbalance.

FUNCTIONAL WEAKNESS IDENTIFICATION

Assessment	Left Brain Score	Right Brain Score	Side of Weakness	Level of Severity
Postural	☐	☐	☐	☐
Vestibular	☐	☐	☐	☐
Auditory	☐	☐	☐	☐
Visual	☐	☐	☐	☐
Proprioception	☐	☐	☐	☐
Tactile	☐	☐	☐	☐
Olfactory	☐	☐	☐	☐

Next, add up the totals from your seven checklists and put them in the appropriate columns. In olfactory and tactile, there is one checklist for hypersensitive and one for hyposensitive. If either of these checklists falls into the abnormal range, then use the lowest number as your guide.

For each list, the lowest possible total score is 10 and the highest possible score is 100. This is what determines the level of severity. The higher the score, the greater the weakness.

A score of 11–40 is Level 3, and a child should start doing exercises at this level.
A score of 41–70 is Level 2.
A score of 71–100 is Level 1.

If the total score in each individual checklist is less than 10, it means that your child most likely does not have a problem in this functional area. He or she will not require or benefit from exercises for this function.

Ideally the Master Hemispheric Checklist, the individual sensory-motor checklists, and the functional assessments should coordinate with one another. If they are not clear-cut, use the Master Hemispheric Checklist to determine the side of the weakness and the individual checklist for each function to determine severity.

The results of the Functional Weakness Identification will be your guide in selecting the type of exercises you will do as part of the Brain Balance Program.

❊ BRAIN BALANCE PROFILE: *Patrick*

OBSESSIVE-COMPULSIVE NO LONGER

The first thing I noticed about Patrick was that he was a pleasant, polite, and very quiet ten-year-old—quite charming, in fact. But his parents were very worried about him.

For most of his short life, Patrick was just a regular boy. He liked to ride his bike and play catch with his dad. His parents were very involved in his activities. The only real complaint they ever had was that Patrick was always a fussy eater. Recently, however, Patrick started acting strangely and was displaying classic signs of obsessive-compulsive disorder. They first noticed it when Patrick started giving the same answer to any question his parents would ask. His response: I'm not sure. Even if he was holding his lunch box in his hand and his mother would ask if he had his lunch, his response would be: I'm not sure.

His parents really got concerned, however, when Patrick started to express almost constant fear, even about things that didn't exist or couldn't possibly happen. His fears of violence started to escalate. For example, one evening while his mother was helping him with his homework, Patrick got highly agitated and frightened. He finally told his mother, a warm and compassionate woman, that he feared she was going to kill him. Eventually his parents came to see me.

Patrick's dad explained that Patrick had always been pretty good at sports but over the past year he had become increasingly clumsy. He could barely catch a ball and had real trouble staying balanced on his bike, even though he used to do these things well. They also said that Patrick had become easily distracted, which had never been a problem before.

When we tested Patrick, we found he had poor motor coordination—he had very bad rhythm and timing and his balance was terrible. He had poor muscle tone and his core stability, in particular, was very bad. Patrick was obviously very intellectual. WIAT testing showed he had a strong vocabulary; nevertheless, he didn't speak much. His WIAT scores put him below his grade level in most of his right brain skills whereas his left brain skills were very high, way above his grade level. His symptoms and his test results concluded that Patrick clearly had a right hemisphere deficiency.

Patrick's parents said he had always been a fussy eater. This clue, plus Patrick's symptoms and how they came on, made us suspect that diet could be the root of his problem. Blood tests revealed he had a number of food intolerances. This really surprised his parents! I explained that food intolerances are different from food allergies. Allergies produce an almost immediate physical response, such as hives or breathing problems. Food intolerances, on the other hand, manifest slowly over several days and cause behavioral symptoms.

We put Patrick on a diet that eliminated all dairy foods and a supplement program. We also implemented sensory, physical, and mental exercises that addressed his right brain deficiency. After one month, Patrick's OCD started to stabilize and he was riding his bicycle with no problem. Over the next several weeks his fears started to wane. Three months later, he was his former self—no fears, no odd behavior, a boy in control of his bike.

WIAT retesting revealed a dramatic increase in right brain activities—on the same level with his left brain skills. His oral expression increased from a second-grade fourth-month level to a twelfth-grade fourth-month level—ten grade levels in three months!

9

SENSORY-MOTOR EXERCISES

Training the Brain Through Physical Stimulation

■

The positive changes that have taken
place in Josh—from being so dysfunctional to an
interacting, happy child—in such a short amount
of time are like a blessed event.

—MARGARET, JOSH'S MOM

■

Now that you have completed the Brain Balance Assessment Program, you are ready to begin the sensory-motor exercises that will get your child on the road to recovery from his or her behavior and learning problems.

Remember, the body and brain are a reciprocal feedback system. Growth of one is dependent on the other, and vice versa. This growth is created by stimulation from the environment. The deficiencies you have identified in your child are the result of the brain not getting the proper stimulation sometime during its course of development.

At first, you will retrain the brain through physical and sensory stimulation. You will gradually notice changes in the problems you have identified through the assessment process. I will then show you how to combine, or integrate, these exercises with mental activities and other forms of stimulation. This is when you will be performing the true Brain Balance Program. As you start implementing the program, you will see the results progress week by week. Altogether, it should take a minimum of about three months to achieve success. It may take longer for lower-functioning children. Keep going until you achieve the desired results.

One thing I always tell parents is not to think of their child as having a learning deficit or behavior problem. Rather, I tell them to think of their child as having a stimulus deficiency. Once this is corrected, *all* the problems you have identified in your child will disappear, or at least significantly improve.

You should find most of these exercises remarkably simple. You will also find that most are very similar to the assessment tests that you have just completed. Even if your child finds some of them difficult to achieve at first, he or she will gradually and continually get better. This I can promise. Just follow them devotedly, keep a positive attitude, and constantly, constantly give your child positive feedback.

It is important to understand that none of these activities will harm your child in any way. There are no negative side effects. If done properly, they can only help your child, strengthening his mind and body, and correcting the brain imbalances that are causing his various symptoms.

Also, keep in mind that genetics as well as current physical ability will play into your child's progress. Some parents will notice more obvious and faster results than others. However, you must also keep in mind that all children have the potential to improve based on consistent use and commitment to the program.

SLOW AND PURPOSEFUL

Throughout the program, you will push your child to the limit but never beyond. Make sure all movements are slow and as purposeful as possible. When you are combining physical movement with mental exercises, the goal is to do it smoothly and in a coordinated fashion.

Read all the directions carefully in order to make sure that you select the correct activity to match your child's hemispheric deficiency and level of competency. You will set priorities as to which exercises to focus on first and then which to integrate into the program as your child progresses.

*   *   *

■ **Reassess, Reassess!** ■

YOU will be able to visibly notice changes in your child as you progress through the Brain Balance Program, but you should make it "official" by periodically redoing the assessment tests in Chapter 8 and recording the results. You should reassess your child once a week while doing the program and once every six months after completion of the program.

Also remember this is just one part of the three-pronged Brain Balance Program. You also will be incorporating an individualized academic and behavioral exercise program, plus a specific diet and nutritional program. Read these sections before you begin, so you can begin incorporating all the changes together. It is important that all are done together, although for most children the skills learned in this chapter are the most valuable in achieving success.   ■

GETTING TO YOUR GOAL

Most of the exercises are divided by function level—Level 1 is the most severe weakness, Level 2 is moderate, and Level 3 is the least severe. You already know where your child fits according to the score you found in Chapter 8.

You will start your child out at his or her current level. The child must be able to do each complete exercise without fault for four consecutive sessions before moving on to the next level. When the child can achieve each exercise without fault at Level 3 for four sessions in a row, you will have successfully completed the program. You may want to periodically repeat these exercises to maintain results, although this is usually not necessary.

BEFORE YOU BEGIN

Before you begin, sit with your child and explain what the two of you are going to do and the benefits he will gain. For example, tell him that he'll get better at athletics, school will get easier, and he'll therefore begin to enjoy being in class more. Explain to him that many, many children have gone through the same program and love the results! Tell him that every child is different so you are going to depend on him to help by interacting with you all the time.

There are three things that can impede progress, so you must continually get feedback from the child. You need to know if:

The movement is too easy or too hard.
The child is having any adverse reactions.
The child is fatigued or getting tired.

Involving the child in all aspects of the program is crucial. Most of their lives, children with FDS have been told what to do. Seldom do people ask them how they are feeling about things.

If the child is young, you can turn it into a game. Joking and humor along the way can help, too. Continually give positive feedback. If you must correct the child, make sure praise follows not too long afterward.

As you progress through the program, you may detect something unusual that you never noticed before and did not become apparent when you were doing the assessments. This should not alarm you. All you need to do is adjust the program by going back one level.

You will be forcing movements that may have been repressed for emotional reasons. These emotions will erupt and should be allowed to surface. Accept it. Also, you may find your child will progress for a time, then regress. This, too, is common. This is not a sign of failure or that something is wrong. Just press on. Continue to encourage and humor him, and keep the humor yourself.

■ It's Win-Win for Parent and Child ■

THE BRAIN Balance Program is a rewarding opportunity for you and your child to interact and share a good time. Disconnected Kids need to feel this connection to their parents. Brain Balance offers you and your child a unique sharing experience. This is especially true of young children. There is no one who can make this happen more than a parent. Each personal interaction you have with your child gives him an additional burst of stimulation, which will only help your child improve even more. It's a win-win environment. Relish it.

■

HEMISPHERIC EXERCISE BASICS

A major key to success is performing these exercises properly. To this end, read these rules, process them, and follow them throughout each and every activity. Always keep in mind:

Frequency is more important than intensity. This means that one quick, short-term burst of energy or effort will not create or maintain changes in the brain. However, changes in the brain will occur with more frequent, less intense types of exercises that are done repeatedly for a set period of time.

Movement must be slow and purposeful. Your child will not be able to focus on the activity if he moves too fast.

Combine with mental activity. If you can combine some form of mental activity with the physical activity (such as jumping rope and reciting the alphabet at the same time), this will help to increase proper stimulation and development of your child's brain. Add these mental activities only at Level 2 or 3 or later on in the program.

Exercises must be performed a minimum of three or four times a week. More is great but less is not recommended. We have found the best success with sticking to the regimen is by keeping it consistent with schooltime. This means weekends off. Besides, kids are most active over the weekend. If they want to also do it over the weekend, that is fine, too.

Do the program after school and before dinner. You will find that your child's appetite will be healthier and her attention span during homework will be better. If you wait until evening, fatigue will become a negative factor.

Stay motivated and positive yourself. Your child is not always going to be enthusiastic about this new routine, but it is imperative that you *always* appear enthusiastic, even if you are tired or feeling discouraged. Your child will more often than not want to do as you do.

Give it time. Remember, there are no short-term, quick-fix types of exercises, but rather exercises and activities that, hopefully, will create a lifestyle change in your child that will make him understand the importance of physical activity as well as mental activity over the course of a lifetime. These lifestyle habits will continue to help increase the capacity of your child's brain, improve its function, and prepare your child for a higher-quality and longer, healthier life!

Proper mind-set is crucial. I can't emphasize enough how important it is that you, as your child's Brain Balance mentor, maintain a positive mind-set. It is very important that you understand and believe that your child's problems are correctable.

You will find many people, including doctors, who will tell you that your child can't improve and that you are wasting your time. If you believe them, then you *will* be wasting your time.

BREATHING AND LARGE MUSCLE EXERCISES

As with any exercise program, Brain Balance requires a little warming up to help loosen muscles and get blood flowing. Breathing exercises and joint mobility are the two exercises that you should have your child do at the beginning of each session.

Besides being good warm-up exercise, they are a crucial part of training the brain to get back in balance.

▶ *The Importance of Proper Breathing*

Most people don't think of breathing as an exercise—but they should. Breathing gives us the oxygen we need to stay alive, but breathing *properly* gives the brain the oxygen it needs to operate at peak capacity. The problem is, most people—kids included—don't get the most out of breathing. Just learning to breathe properly can make a world of difference to children with FDS.

Breathing is integral to any exercise regimen. It is the foundation of practices such as yoga, transcendental meditation, and certain religious rites aimed at increasing mental focus and attention—including the Brain Balance Program.

Oddly enough, the type of breathing that is most beneficial is the breathing we observe in babies. It's called diaphragmatic breathing, or belly breathing. If you watch a baby breathe, you will see the belly go up and down. But the majority of people lose that instinct early on and start to breathe using the chest. Diaphragmatic breathing takes conscious effort at first, but children can adapt to it easily. Your child may start out doing it for only a short period, but if you keep reminding him, this can change over time.

▶ *Diaphragmatic Breathing*

⟷ Both hemispheres

⟷ All levels

Have your child stand straight and tall with her arms at her sides. Ask the child to keep her lips pursed and inhale deeply and slowly through the nose. Count the number of seconds it takes. Then tell her to open her mouth and exhale even slower until all the air is expelled from the lungs. This should take twice as long as the inhale. Count the number of seconds it takes for inhalation and then have the child attempt to exhale (breathe out) through her mouth for twice as long, releasing the air in a slow, controlled fashion. This will have the child breathe more deeply and slowly from the diaphragm as opposed to the chest. Repeat three to five times. Also, repeat this breathing routine intermittently throughout her planned exercise schedule.

The goal over time is to slowly increase the time on both inhalation and exhalation. Encourage your child to do this exercise throughout her day, especially when she's feeling anxious, stressed, or restless. For example, if you see her looking anxious or agitated, say, "Now stop and take a slow deep breath, just like we practiced. Now let it out even slower." Train her to think to do this in school and other settings when you can't be there to remind her.

▶ *Joint Mobility and Flexibility Exercise*

Moving the large muscles and joints—what we call postural muscle activity—is extremely important because it provides the majority of stimulation that the brain needs to get back in sync. However, it is also an important warm-up exercise because stretching helps increase mobility and flexibility in the joints and muscles, which in turn improves their ability to stimulate the brain. It also contributes to making the exercises in the rest of the program easier.

You will assist your child in stretching by gently pulling on his arms and legs. You are not to pull hard or put a lot of pressure on the joints when doing this.

These exercises will distract and stretch the spinal muscles as well as help to stretch and increase pressure on the spinal joints and ligaments.

At the same time you will also be stretching and stimulating the joints in the arms and legs.

▶ *Proprioceptive Joint Distraction Exercises*

    ⟷ Both hemispheres
    ⟷ All levels

This is a whole body exercise designed to help center or calm the child while simultaneously increasing brain stimulation. You'll want to use a mat, a soft blanket, or a towel.

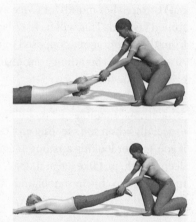

Have your child lie facedown on the floor with feet extended and arms straight out next to the head. Grasp the child's wrists and gently pull. Hold 5 seconds and release. Repeat six times, waiting 5 to 10 seconds between each stretch.

Ask your child to turn over on his belly and extend his hands straight out overhead. Grasp his ankles and gently pull. Hold 5 seconds and release. Repeat six times, waiting 5 to 10 seconds between each stretch.

> ▼ **CAUTION:** Make sure that you pull gently and slowly. Be very careful not to stretch forcefully. If the child becomes agitated, stop, calm him down, then resume.

> ▼ **TIP:** If your child is hypersensitive to touch, use prolonged, firm touch rather than quick, light touch. Limit the amount of touching and always alert your child before you are ready to touch him.

RESTORING SENSORY DEFICITS

As I demonstrated several times in Part 1, there is a link between abnormal behavior and sensory deficits—smell, touch, vision, hearing, and balance.

It has often been assumed that these deficits are static and cannot be changed or improved. Nothing is further from the truth.

OLFACTORY (SMELLING) EXERCISES

In almost all the children I work with, especially those with right hemisphere deficits, we have found a functional deficit in the sense of smell.

We have found and studies also show that when the sense of smell is improved through training, problems associated with the deficit automatically correct themselves. When we perform smell exercises similar to the ones I am about to show you, we see a significant, if not complete, return of the sense of smell in 90 percent of the cases. As a result, we also see a change in eating habits. Children become open to new and varied foods. They no longer judge food by its appearance or feel. This, in turn, leads to a healthier diet, which provides the brain with the nutrients and energy it needs to build and grow new areas of the brain. As I explained earlier, this is often associated with a positive change in nonverbal communication, emotional awareness of self and others, immune regulation, digestion, and body/spatial awareness.

▶ *Smell Distance Detection Exercise*

→ Right hemisphere weakness: Stimulate right nostril only.
→ Use strong scents such as:

Black pepper
Burnt wood
Coffee
Eucalyptus
Fish oil
Lemon
Lime
Mustard
Onion
Peppermint

← Left hemisphere weakness: Stimulate left nostril only.

← Use pleasant scents such as:

Apple
Banana
Cherry
Chocolate
Grape
Lavender
Orange
Pineapple
Rose
Strawberry

Just as you did in the assessment test, tell your child that you are going to play the smell game. Explain that he can't peek so he needs to be blindfolded, and that he has to guess each scent. You will need nine different canisters for nine different scents. You should vary the canisters and use different scents so your child cannot anticipate what may be coming next. You can vary the strength—make them strong sometimes and weaker at others. Do a test exercise first. Always let your child know if he is guessing correctly or not.

With the child blindfolded, ask him to press one nostril closed with his finger or do it for him. Hold the first canister about 12 inches from the nostril. Ask if he can detect a smell. If he can't, move an inch closer and ask again. Continue until he can detect the smell. When he can, ask him to name the scent. If he does not get it right, give him two more chances. If it is difficult for him, you can offer three or four choices.

▼ **TIP:** Each day after the game, take a little essential oil and place it on the collar of his shirt under the nostril that you are stimulating. Vary the smell each day as much as possible. Do not place oil directly on skin as this may burn or irritate.

Level 1 goal: Three correct smells in a row.
Level 2 goal: Six correct in a row.
Level 3 goal: Nine correct in a row.

If the goal is achieved without any mistakes for four days in a row, move to the next level. When your child gets nine smells in a row correct for four days in a row at Level 3, you have achieved success. Your child's smell should be back in sync and his sense of smell will continue to improve on its own from this point on. Periodically, however, repeat "the game" to make sure your child can still pass the sniff test.

▼ **TIP:** Some children have such an impaired sense of smell that they can't sniff correctly. If this is the case, demonstrate how to do it and work with him until he gets it right.

VISION EXERCISES

It is well documented that altering the color of a visual stimulus improves areas of the brain that govern cognitive, behavioral, autonomic, immune, and emotional functions. It has also been found that the two hemispheres of the brain respond differently to different colors. The color red, for example, inhibits right hemisphere activity and enhances left brain activity, which is why altering color through the use of lenses or colored acetate, as you will do in this exercise, enhances reading ability.

These vision exercises work because of the way receptors send light to the brain. Larger visual receptors located in the retina and the outer periphery of the eye are more sensitive to certain frequencies of light waves. This makes them more sensitive to higher-frequency colors or light waves that literally move faster.

There are seven primary colors based on seven different frequencies of light waves in the visual light spectrum.

The lowest frequency is red, which increases to orange, yellow, green, blue, indigo, and the highest, violet. Green is the middle frequency.

The lower-frequency colors are more specific to the left hemisphere because the receptors that send information to the left hemisphere are sensitive to more detailed but also slower-moving light waves. So, anything that will increase speed in the left hemisphere and inhibit the right hemisphere will enhance the left brain's ability to hear and read words.

Using an eye patch also enhances reading ability. It helps strengthen eye muscles, and children with FDS have weak eye muscles in the dysfunctional side of the brain. Studies show that wearing an eye patch can also improve reading skills in children who do not have weak eye muscles because covering one eye increases stimulation in the eye that is reading.

These exercises use both techniques for visual improvement in three areas: light stimulation, fast and slow tracking, and convergence/divergence.

▶ *The Brain Balance Way*

They are similar to the visual assessment tests you are already familiar with. The only difference is that you will be directing the exercises to only one eye with some of these activities.

▶ *Pencil Push-Ups*

→ ← Right and left hemisphere deficiency

Do these exercises if your child showed an inability to cross her eyes to the proper distance in the assessment test. This inability is characteristic of a right hemisphere weakness. However, if the left eye is weak or tired out during testing, then it might show a left hemisphere weakness. Either way, improving the strength, endurance, and coordination of both eyes will help to balance a weakness in either side of the brain. As you did in the assessment, explain to the child what you are going to do before you perform the test.

Have the child stand or sit relaxed, with the head straight and steady. Hold a pencil approximately 18 inches in front of her nose. She should be able to focus and see only one pencil at this distance. If she sees two, move the pencil back inch by inch until she sees only one. Slowly bring the pencil toward the nose and tell her to let you know the moment she sees the pencil double. Stop and note the distance. Ask her to try as hard as possible to see it as one pencil again. If she can do this, continue to slowly bring the pencil closer to her nose until she tells you that she sees two images again. Repeat your instructions as before. Continue to bring the pencil closer to the nose until she can no longer get rid of the double image. At this point, have her concentrate her attention on the pencil as you slowly back the pencil away from the nose to the original starting position. Encourage her to follow the pencil and stare at it the whole way out. Repeat the entire exercise three times if she does not get too tired.

As the eye muscles get stronger and more coordinated, you will notice that the pencil will remain as one as you get closer and closer to the nose. You should be able to get within an inch or two of the nose without double vision. This is the goal.

Level 1: Do the exercise fully one time.
Level 2: Do the exercise fully two times.
Level 3: Do the exercise at least three times.

Other options: This is a tough exercise. Try it yourself and you will see how tired your eyes get after just one time. In young children, I have found that it is sometimes easier if you use a penlight or a small round mirror or reflective surface. This helps a child focus better; besides, children love seeing their own image. Do the exercise exactly as you would with the pencil, asking instead, *"How many of you do you see?"*

▼ **HINT:** If the child doesn't respond, then simply watch her eyes. If the child looks away or if one eye turns out, you can assume she is seeing double.

▶ *Fast Tracking Exercise*

→ Right hemisphere deficiency: Majority of exercises to the left direction.
← Left hemisphere deficiency: Majority of exercises to the right direction.

When you did this as an assessment test, the goal was to determine if the eyes were not moving quickly enough, which resulted in either overshooting or undershooting a moving target (your finger).

In this exercise, you will use fast movements and concentrate these movements on the slower side—that is, the side that overshoots the target. But the activity must be random for the exercise to work properly. This means that you will exercise both eyes, only you will be exercising the weak side more often. For example, in a series of ten movements, three will be to the strong side and seven to the weak side. Make sure that the child moves both eyes quickly to both sides. This is enough of a balance to keep the child guessing, but it will work one side significantly more than the other.

Have the child stand or sit, relaxed, head straight and facing you at eye level. Tell him that you are going to wiggle a finger and you want him to look at your finger quickly without moving his head. Tell him when you say "Okay," he should look back at your nose. For a child with a right brain weakness, wiggle your right finger seven times and your left finger three. Do it vice versa for a left hemisphere weakness. Continually mix this up so the child doesn't know which finger will wiggle next. Take note if the child is overshooting by counting how many times he misses the target. You will know this because the child will move the eyes in two steps to get to the target instead of one. Each time mark down how many times he misses.

As the child improves, he will get faster and more accurate with his eye movements until the two eyes are equal.

> ▼ **HINT:** To increase concentration and improve the effect, you can wear a colored glove or tie a small ribbon or string on one finger. Use a blue ribbon or string on the right finger and a red one on the left finger. This will make it more interesting and the colors are specific to the side of the brain you wish to stimulate.

← Left Brain Colors	→ Right Brain Colors
Red	Blue
Orange	Indigo
Yellow	Violet

▶ *Slow Tracking Exercise (Pursuit)*

→ Right hemisphere weakness: Exercise right direction only.
← Left hemisphere weakness: Exercise left direction only.

In the slow eye tracking assessment test, you found the deficiency by identifying the side that the eyes were having more difficulty moving toward. In correcting the deficiency, you will only slow track in the weak direction (toward the weak hemisphere).

Stand in front of your child and move a few steps from center and farthest from the side that your finger will start. (If you are working with the right brain, you will move to the left of center.) You want to stand as far away as possible as the eyes can turn. Hold up your index finger or a pencil about 12 inches back from her face and ask your child to keep her head straight and turn her eyes toward your finger. Tell her she should not move her head. Ask her to follow your finger or the pencil with her eyes as you slowly move from far left to far right. Ask her to close her eyes. Go back to your original position. Ask the child to open her eyes and locate your finger. Do the exercise again and repeat for a total of ten times. Go slowly enough so the child can follow. If she loses the finger or her eyes jump, you are going too fast. Slow down. If the child loses interest, she blinks excessively, or the eyes jump, stop. As you continue to do this exercise on a daily basis, she will start to improve.

For Level 1, start with slow movements until the child can do the exercise with no jumping.

Then progress to fast-tracking movements. When he can do this easily without overshooting the target, then repeat all exercises two times. When he can do this without any jumping or overshooting four sessions in a row, you have reached your goal. Move to the next level for the next session.

Level 1: Do only slow movements.
Level 2: Do slow and fast tracking.
Level 3: Do all tracking movements fully two times.

▼ **TIP:** Make sure that you always ask your child to close her eyes at the end of each slow tracking movement. This is an important step because it helps focus light toward the weak side.

▼ **HINT:** As in the previous exercise, you can use a colored glove or ribbon. Blue for right hemisphere weakness; red for left.

▶ Light-Blocking Activities

→ Right brain deficiency: Block the right eye.
← Left brain deficiency: Block the left eye.

This exercise is a very powerful stimulus because it blocks light in an unbalanced fashion. It stimulates one hemisphere while taking away stimulation from the other hemisphere. It is an especially good approach for children who are hypersensitive to light.

. . .

Level 1: Eye Patch

This step involves the child wearing an eye patch. Children usually tolerate this well. Some even think it's a lot of fun if you make it a game.

This exercise is simple. Have your child wear the patch over the eye that is on the side of the weak hemisphere. Start with 30 minutes and progress to 2 hours of continual use. As the child's tolerance increases, have him wear it to watch TV or play on the computer. Then have the child wear the patch to read. For children with a left hemisphere deficiency, it should help make reading easier. When the child is ready (he can tolerate this for 2 full hours), he is ready to go to Level 2 and replace the patch with blocking glasses.

▼ **CAUTION:** Keep an eye on your child as he may lose his balance or misjudge distance at first until he gets used to wearing a patch and blocking glasses.

Level 2: Blocking Glasses
→ Right brain deficiency: Block right half of both lenses.
← Left brain deficiency: Block left half of both lenses.

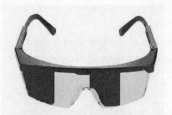

Hemifield glasses are special lenses that can be manipulated to partially block light from entering the retina. They are easy to make on your own. Buy a small pair of safety goggles, or even swimming goggles for smaller children, with clear lenses that wrap around the side of the face. You can find them at any home or hardware store. Make sure they fit your child's head securely. To get the blocking effect, use paint, White-Out, or masking tape to completely cover half the lenses as illustrated and specified above. This means you will be blocking the outside of one lens and the inside of the other. On the outer block, make sure you block the lens all the way around the side. The intent of wearing these glasses is to help balance brain activity.

Introduce these glasses to your child by telling her that these are special glasses that will make school or sports easier. Start out by having your child wear the glasses for a half hour a day, then build up to a longer time, optimally 2 hours of continual use. Have your child wear these glasses when watching TV or using the computer. Don't make your child wear them when doing homework unless she wants to do so. After she tolerates this for 2 hours, your child will be ready for Level 3, light stimulation.

> ▼ **HINT:** If you get resistance about wearing blocking glasses, tell your child that she can only watch TV or use the computer if she wears them. It is important that you do not back down! (You'll find out why when you read Chapter 12.)

LEVEL 3: LIGHT STIMULATION

In this exercise you will use light to stimulate the eye by making the eyes constrict. You will need a penlight or a small flashlight set on the lowest setting. If the light is too bright (causing the child to turn his head), tape a penny over the center of the lens or cover it with a piece of clear colored acetate. Use a color that coordinates with the hemispheric deficiency from the list on page 162.

Have the child put on the blocking glasses. With the flashlight ready, ask the child to look straight ahead in the distance. Position yourself and the light about 6 to 8 inches away from the eye to the side opposite the child's hemisphere deficiency—that is, to the child's left side if she has a right brain deficiency, and to the right for a left brain deficiency. Turn the flashlight on and shine it into the corner of the eye closer to you. This will make the pupils of both eyes constrict and then dilate. Count how long it takes for this to happen. When the eye stops dilating, you can stop.

As you do this in each session, it will take longer and longer for dilation to occur. You want the eyes to stay constricted a long time—approximately 10 to 15 seconds is ideal. This is a normal light response. If your child turns away and is extremely sensitive, discontinue the exercise and try again tomorrow.

THE THERAPEUTIC USE OF SOUND AND LIGHT

Music (sound) and color (light) therapy for health and healing can be traced all the way back to ancient civilizations but it wasn't until the last half of the twentieth century that Western medicine started to embrace it for its ability to promote positive change in the body. Music and color work by radiating genuine energy frequencies. Auditory and visual stimulation, through the use of sound and light, has a therapeutic effect because of the different frequencies at which it functions.

Color (light) is a powerful stimulus. We are susceptible to its influences even though we are not consciously aware of it. For example, looking at bright red, or even wearing it, can elicit different emotional, autonomic, or motor responses. Being in a room painted blue or wearing blue can elicit these same effects.

Sound, like light, is based on wave length and frequencies. Just as the visible light spectrum is broken into seven primary light frequencies or colors, audible sound is broken up into seven primary sound frequencies or notes. This is not coincidental. It is based on the fact that the brain processes hearing and vision in a similar fashion.

The two hemispheres of the brain process sound and light differently, based on the frequency (speed) of the stimulus. Up to a certain point, sound and light follow a parallel path and then they separate. Light, the faster-moving stimulus that carries less detailed information, goes primarily to the right hemisphere. Sound, the faster, higher-frequency stimulus with more detailed information, goes to the left hemisphere. With sound, however, the lower-frequency sounds also transfer less-detailed information. This slower-frequency sound is transmitted to the right hemisphere. Higher frequency—that is, faster more rapidly changing sounds (such as speech)—is processed primarily by the left hemisphere. The different frequencies of both light and sound cause brain cells to fire at different speeds.

■ Color and Sound Relationships ■

ACCORDING to the theory of color and music, there are comparable vibrational frequencies between the seven spectrum colors and the seven-note scale (including whole tones and half tones).

Red vibrates to middle C = Red stimulates the left brain, middle C stimulates the right.

Orange to D = Orange stimulates the left brain, D stimulates the right.

Yellow to E = Yellow stimulates the left brain, E stimulates the right.

Green to F (half step) = Green stimulates the right brain, F stimulates the right.

Blue to G = Blue stimulates the right brain, G stimulates the left.

Indigo to A = Indigo stimulates the right brain, A stimulates the left.

Violet to B = Violet stimulates the right brain, B stimulates the left.

The seven pure spectrum colors relate to the middle octave of the keyboard. However, there are continuing relationships between the treble (higher) and bass (lower) octaves with various shading of the spectrum colors. The colors relating to the octave below the middle octave would be deeper and darker, but with the same tonal correlation. For example, the C below the middle C would still be in the red family, but would be deeper than the red of middle C. The tones above the middle octave would be represented by lighter and more luminous colors.

Sound in the form of music has a very powerful effect on brain activity. We have all experienced how music can evoke memories and emotions. Think of a sad scene in a movie. When music moves in over the scene, it accentuates the emotion (and often brings on your tears). The emotion is actually driven by the sound frequency and other qualities associated with the music and the side of the brain in which the sound in processed. For sad scenes, this would be the right brain. Of course, music can just as easily evoke positive and motivational emotions.

MUSICAL BRAIN BALANCE ACTIVITIES

→ Right hemisphere = Low-frequency sound
← Left hemisphere = High-frequency sound

The different qualities that make one musical piece different from another are processed in different sides of the brain. In the following exercises, you will have your child listen to music that most accentuates the musical qualities that are processed in his or her deficient brain hemisphere as follows:

▶ *Right Hemisphere*

Harmony
Interval
Quality
Timbre
Spatial, temporal, and long-term patterns

▶ *Left Hemisphere*

Rapid variance in volume
Pitch
Timing
Rhythm
Lyrics
Familiar sounds

Unfortunately, you can't go to a store and purchase music that is purely left hemisphere or right hemisphere. It doesn't exist. There is a tremendous amount of research documenting what types of music and which frequencies of sounds affect either sides of the brain, but no one has ever taken this research and formulated music based on this information.

When I became aware of this, I contacted an individual who is both a composer and a musician. Together we arranged various pieces of music that are designed specifically to affect each hemisphere. We use these compositions, which are branded as Brain Balance Music, to work with children in our Brain Balance Centers. Other professionals also have been using Brain Balance Music and are getting outstanding results. Information on how to purchase Brain Balance Music can be found on page 261. Though I believe this music is the best option, there are other choices.

If you are familiar with musical tones, you can choose your own based on the qualities described above that are specific to your child's deficiency. If not, here is a list of selections from which you can choose. Remember, music and color are the opposite in the brain. For example, red music is low frequency—the music goes to the right brain but the color goes to the left. However, we refer to it as red music because both color and sound have the same frequency.

▶ *Right Brain Music: Note C (Red)*

CLASSICAL
"March Militaire," by Schubert
Any march by John Philip Sousa
"Sailor's Dance" from *The Red Poppy Ballet Suite,* by Reinhold Gliére

NEW AGE
"Mars," from *The Planets,* by Gustav Holst

"On the Edge," by Mickey Hart
"Diga Rhythm," by Mickey Hart

▶ *Right Brain Music: Note D (Orange)*

CLASSICAL
Hungarian Dance No. 5, by Brahms
"Habanera," from *Carmen*, by Bizet
"Capriccio Espagnole", by Rimsky-Korsakov

NEW AGE
"Winterfall Music," by Paul Warner
"Jupiter," from *The Planets*, by Gustav Holst
"Eagle's Call," by Bruce Hurnow

▶ *Right Brain Music: Note E (Yellow)*

CLASSICAL
"Arabeske," by Schumann
"Fountains of Rome," by Respighi
Piano Concerto No. 26, by Mozart

NEW AGE
"Lemurian Sunrise," by Paul Lloyd Warner
"Dawn," by Steven Halpern
"Kitaro Ki," by Kitaro

▶ *Right Brain Music: Note F (Green)*

CLASSICAL
Melody in F, by Rubinstein
Violin Concerto in E Minor, by Mendelssohn
"Claire de Lune," by Debussy

NEW AGE
"Pan Flute," by La Mir
"Ocean," by Larkin
"Fairy Ring," by Mike Rowland

•   •   •

▶ *Left Brain Music: Note G (Blue)*

CLASSICAL
Air on a G String, by Bach
"Ave Maria," by Schubert
"The Swan," by Saint-Saëns

NEW AGE
"Divine Gypsy," by Paramahansa Yogananda
"Crystal Cave," from *Back to Atlantis,* by Upper Astral
Vocal selection: "Be Still," by Rosemary Crow

▶ *Left Brain Music: Note B (Indigo)*

CLASSICAL
"Traumerei," by Schumann
"Adagio," from Symphony No. 1 in C Minor, by Brahms
"Poéme for Violin and Orchestra," by Ernest Chausson

NEW AGE
"Angel Love," by Aeoliah
"Inside," by Paul Horn
"Venus," from *The Planets,* by Holst

▶ *Left Brain Music: Note A (Violet)*

CLASSICAL
Piano Concerto in B Minor, by Tchaikovsky
Liebestraum, by Liszt
Gregorian Chants

NEW AGE
"The Great Pyramid," by Paul Horn
"Neptune," from *The Planets,* by Gustav Holst
"Eventide," by Stephen Halpern

Source: From *Healing with Music and Color: A Beginner's Guide,* by Mary Bassano (Samuel Wesier, Inc., 1992).

▶ *Sound-Blocking Exercise*

→ Right hemisphere deficiency: Block right ear.
← Left hemisphere deficiency: Block left ear.

These exercises involve using an earplug in one ear to block sound. Blocking the music in the "good" ear will allow natural sound to enter and stimulate the brain without affecting the other side and overstimulating the child with sound.

> ▼ **TIP:** You will only need to use one earplug but you will have to purchase a set (they are inexpensive), which you can find at any pharmacy. I like to use the type that is soft and malleable because it is comfortable in a child's ear. These plugs also come in bright colors, so kids love to wear them.

You can use any musical selection as long as it is specific to your child's hemispheric weakness. You do not have to use music. Natural sound can have the same effect. You can do a combination of the two.

Ideally, you should have your child use the earplug and blocking lenses at the same time. You can still achieve success using them separately, but when they are combined, the effect can be extremely powerful. If doing the two at the same time is too much for your child, do them each on alternating days.

As with the blocking lenses, start out by having the child wear the earplug while watching TV or using the computer. The beauty of using Brain Balance Music is that even if the child refuses to wear an earplug or pulls it out, the music is still specifically designed to stimulate one side of the brain more than the other.

How long you need to use an earplug will in large part depend on your child's tolerance level. Small children can pull an earplug out within a few minutes. Older, higher-functioning children should be able to keep it in as long as you want. Ideally you should start with about 30 minutes and build up to 60 minutes at a time.

Level 1

You'll start out just having your child get used to wearing an earplug. Have your child wear one earplug in the appropriate ear for a minimum of 30 minutes. When he can do this without fussing or pulling it out for four sessions in a row, you are ready to move on to Level 2.

LEVEL 2

Select music that corresponds to your child's deficiency from the list on pages 168–170. Plug your child's ear and put the music in your CD player. Play the music ambiently so your child does not have to wear any headphones at first. Make sure it is a comfortable volume for the child. Your child does not have to be actively listening to get the proper effect, but he must be within hearing distance of the music. Play the music while you're driving him in the car, when he is at the computer, or when he is just hanging around the house playing. Start out at 10 minutes a day and build up to 30 minutes. Note how long he listens without making a fuss.

LEVEL 3

For this exercise you will not need an earplug but you will need headphones. An inexpensive set will suffice. Make sure the headphones fit comfortably on the child's head. Remove the earpiece from the side of your child's "good" ear so the sound only goes to the side of the deficiency.

Use the same time progression and criteria as you did for Level 2. Gradually increase the time until your child can tolerate an hour straight.

VESTIBULAR EXERCISES

▶ Level 1: Slow Spinning

Have the child sit straight in the chair with the head bent slightly forward. Legs must be off the floor and on the chair, either tucked in or Indian style. Instruct the child to keep the head still during the exercise. Start spinning the chair slowly to make sure the child can tolerate the exercise. You only need to do this for a minute. Ask the child to close his eyes and very slowly spin the chair. It should take 60 seconds to do one full rotation. While you are spinning, instruct the child to point a finger in the direction he is spinning. Also, tell him to let you know when you've stopped spinning the chair. Slowly bring the chair to a stop. Ask the child if he is still spinning. If he says yes, then ask him to tell you when he stops. Once the child says the spinning stopped, have him open his eyes. Ask if he feels dizzy or sick. Then repeat the same exercise in the opposite direction. Note if the child can correctly identify the direction of the motion, when he said the chair stopped spinning, and if he felt dizzy when he opened his eyes. Record the results of both scores. You will continue to do this until the child no longer gets dizzy and he can accurately name the direction he is moving in for four sessions.

▶ *Level 2: Fast Spinning*

→ Right hemisphere deficiency: Spin clockwise (right).
← Left hemisphere deficiency: Spin counterclockwise (left).

Start from the same position as before. With her eyes open, spin the child in the direction as specified above ten times. Each rotation should take 2 seconds. This should make the child dizzy. At the end of the tenth rotation, stop the child, stand off to the side, have the child look at the ceiling, and quickly look at her eyes. You should see both eyes going back and forth briskly. Count how long this continues. When the eyes stop moving, the dizziness should be gone. Stay at Level 2 until the eyes shake back and forth for 6 seconds. When this happens for four sessions in a row, move to Level 3.

▶ *Level 3*

Repeat Level 2 and continue until eye movement and dizziness last for 15 seconds.

PROPRIOCEPTIVE EXERCISES

If you had never heard of proprioceptivity before picking up this book, you know what it is all about now. In essence, it is what Functional Disconnection Syndrome is all about. Because most children with FDS do not feel their bodies very well, they have low muscle tone, especially in the big, core muscles that provide stability. These muscles also provide the vast majority of subconscious stimulation to the brain. All these exercises are designed to improve balance and stability and to increase muscle tone so a child can react more quickly.

▶ *Level 1: One Foot in Front of the Other*

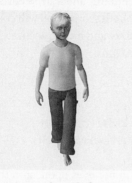

Before starting this exercise, have the child remove his shoes and one sock. Have him remove the left sock if you want to stimulate the right hemisphere; remove the right sock if you are trying to stimulate the left. Ask the child to stand straight, eyes open, with feet together, and move one foot directly in front of the other, as shown in the illustration. The goal is for the child to remain still without falling or leaning to the side for 30 seconds. Be close at hand to catch the child in case he falls. When he can do this for four sessions in a row, move to Level 2.

▶ *Level 2: One Leg Stand*

→ Right hemisphere deficiency: Bend right knee.
← Left hemisphere deficiency: Bend left knee.

Have the child stand facing you with legs together and eyes open. Ask him to bend his leg as specified above and remain still as long as possible. The goal is for the child to remain still in this position for 30 seconds. When he can do this for four sessions in a row, go to Level 3.

▶ *Level 3: One Leg Stand*

Take the same position as Level 2 but with eyes closed. When the child can remain perfectly still for 30 seconds for four sessions in a row, he has achieved his goal.

▶ *Supine Bridge Core Exercises*

LEVEL 1

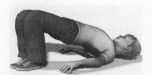

Have the child lie on her back with knees bent and feet flat on the floor shoulder width apart. Hands should be straight at the sides for support. Help the child get off the ground by lifting her backside off the floor so that the spine is straight, as if forming a bridge. Do this exercise at each session until she can remain still in this position for 30 seconds. In older children, the goal is 60 seconds.

Level 2

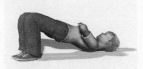

Have the child get in the same position as in Level 1 but have him cross his arms across his chest. This takes away some of their stability and adds resistance to their muscles, making it harder to maintain the position. Have the child get in the bridge position as in Level 1. When he can maintain this position without buckling or moving for 60 seconds four sessions in a row, move to Level 3.

Level 3

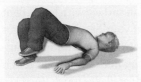

Have the child assume the same position as Level 1 and get into the bridge position. Ask him to raise one leg off the ground about an inch or two and maintain this position for as long as possible, up to 30 seconds. Switch legs and repeat. The goal is to do this exercise until he can remain still in both positions without moving for 30 seconds for four sessions in a row.

▶ Prone Bridge Core Stability Exercise

Level 1

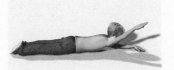

Have the child lie down flat on her belly on the floor with arms straight out in front above her head. Ask the child to raise her head and one arm off the floor and keep the arm perfectly straight. Have her hold this position for as long as possible up to 15 seconds. Repeat with the opposite arm and each leg. The goal is to achieve this position on both sides for 15 seconds. When she can do this four sessions in a row, move to Level 2.

LEVEL 2

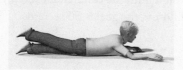

Repeat the same exercise as in Level 1 but aim for 30 seconds off the floor in both positions. When the child achieves this for four sessions in a row, move to Level 3.

LEVEL 3

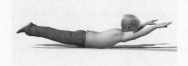

Assume the same position as in Levels 1 and 2. Ask the child to lift all four limbs off the floor for as long as possible. The goal is to hold this position steady for 60 seconds four sessions in a row.

▶ Curl-Ups (or Partial Curl-Ups)

Have the child lie on a flat cushioned and clean surface with knees bent and feet about 12 inches from his backside. Put your hands over his feet for support. Ask him to cross his arms and place his palms on his shoulders. Now ask him to raise his trunk and curl up until his elbows touch his thighs. Ask him to lie back down so the shoulder blades touch the floor, for one curl-up. Continue to do this for 1 minute while counting aloud. The goal is to do this fluidly without error for the number of times appropriate for their age and sex in 1 minute.

LEVEL 1

GOALS FOR BOYS AND GIRLS
Ages 4–7: 15 curl-ups
Ages 8–12: 25 curl-ups
Ages 13–17: 35 curl-ups

LEVEL 2

GOALS FOR BOYS
Ages 4–7: 25 curl-ups
Ages 8–12: 35 curl-ups
Ages 13–17: 45 curl-ups

GOALS FOR GIRLS
Ages 4–7: 25 curl-ups
Ages 8–12: 35 curl-ups
Ages 13–17: 40 curl-ups

LEVEL 3
GOALS FOR BOYS
Ages 4–7: 35 curl-ups
Ages 8–12: 45 curl-ups
Ages 13–17: 55 curl-ups

GOALS FOR GIRLS
Ages 4–7: 35 curl-ups
Ages 8–12: 45 curl-ups
Ages 13–17: 50 curl-ups

▶ *Right-Angle Push-Ups*

Have the child lie facedown on the floor in the classic push-up position: hands under shoulders, fingers straight, and legs straight, parallel, and slightly apart with the toes supporting the feet. Ask the child to push up, keeping the back and knees straight, and then lower the body until there is a 90-degree angle at the elbows. Place your hand flat underneath her chest so when she comes back down to the floor, she touches your hand before pushing up again. The entire exercise should take 3 seconds. The goal is to do this fluidly without error for the number of times appropriate for their age and sex.

LEVEL 1
GOALS FOR BOYS
Ages 4–7: 5 push-ups
Ages 8–12: 10 push-ups
Ages 13–17: 15 push-ups

GOALS FOR GIRLS
Ages 4–7: 5 push-ups
Ages 8–12: 10 push-ups
Ages 13–17: 15 push-ups

Level 2

GOALS FOR BOYS
Ages 4–7: 5 push-ups
Ages 8–12: 15 push-ups
Ages 13–17: 30 push-ups

GOALS FOR GIRLS
Ages 4–7: 5 push-ups
Ages 8–12: 10 push-ups
Ages 13–17: 15 push-ups

Level 3

GOALS FOR BOYS
Ages 4–7: 15 push-ups
Ages 8–12: 25 push-ups
Ages 13–17: 45 push-ups

GOALS FOR GIRLS
Ages 4–7: 15 push-ups
Ages 8–12: 20 push-ups
Ages 13–17: 25 push-ups

TACTILE EXERCISES

→ Right hemisphere deficiency: Brush left side.
← Left hemisphere deficiency: Brush right side.

There are no levels for this first activity.

▶ *Tactile Desensitization Activity*

With a small soft brush, lightly brush the inside of the forearm and then the leg above the knee of the appropriate side. Brush only the arm and the leg opposite the side of the hemisphere you wish to stimulate; for example, left arm and leg only for a right brain weakness. Repeat ten times at the beginning of each tactile exercise session.

▶ *Number Tracing Exercise*

Demonstrate this exercise prior to doing it. Use a form of the numbers the child will be able to recognize. For example, if he writes the number 4, do not use a *4*.

LEVEL 1

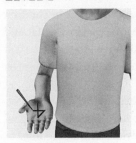

With eyes covered, have the child sit with arms outstretched and palms up. With the eraser end of a pencil, trace a digit from 0 to 9 on the appropriate arm and ask him to identify the number. Do this a total of three times with three different numbers. When he can do the exercises accurately for four sessions, move on to Level 2.

LEVEL 2

Repeat Level 1 but write six random numbers. When he gets it accurate three times in a row, proceed to Level 3.

LEVEL 3

Repeat Level 1 but write nine random numbers. When he gets it accurate three times in a row, you have reached your goal.

AEROBIC EXERCISES

In 1999 a California scientist made an amazing finding: Rats that ran on a treadmill for 12 days in a row doubled their number of brain cells. This was considered such an astounding finding at the time that the Salk Institute researchers who made the discovery all took up running.

We now know that, like rats, humans have the ability to reproduce brain cells through aerobic activity. (The process is called neurogenesis.) If adults and rats can create new brain cells, imagine the possibility for a developing child's brain!

•   •   •

▶ Aerobic Exercises for Children

The link between aerobic exercise and brain growth is oxygen. Aerobics pump oxygen into the body. This increased supply is of the utmost importance in Brain Balance. In research studies as well as in our own program, childhood activities such as running, biking, jumping jacks, jumping rope, and so forth, have proven to be highly effective in decreasing hyperactivity as well as increasing focus and concentration in children diagnosed with ADHD (not to mention the positive cardiovascular and overall effects on the body). As part of the Brain Balance Program, you will have your child do an aerobic activity at least three to four times a week but preferably every day.

Here are effective activities that children particularly enjoy. Switch them around to give your child variety and keep her interested. The goal is for your child to do aerobics for increasing periods of time in order to increase his or her endurance and overall oxygenation to the brain. As is the goal of Brain Balance, many of these exercises inherently include some form of functional integration. For example, jumping rope integrates aerobic activity with coordination, rhythm, and timing, which requires mental focus. Try to integrate some form of mental exercise (as described previously) with the aerobic exercise.

▶ Running in Place

Mark an X on the floor or somewhere outdoors on your property with a piece of tape. Demonstrate for your child how to run in place, moving the arms and legs. Remember, controlled movement is very important so offer guidance to the child as needed. Start with 1 minute followed by a 1-minute rest. Slowly increase the time 1 minute at a time.

Only increase the time when the child can run in place smoothly with her arms and legs moving in good rhythm.

As the child is able, have her perform the exercise with her eyes closed.

Again, as your child improves, continue to integrate mental exercises such as saying the alphabet, numerical operations, or even making up a story verbally with the aerobic exercise.

·   ·   ·

▶ Jumping

Have your child jump up and down on the X for a period of 30 seconds, followed by a 30-second rest. Increase the time in increments of 30 seconds as the child is able.

▶ Minitrampoline

Children find a trampoline fun (and it saves wear and tear on your floor). Since controlled movement is the key, mark an X in the center of the trampoline and have the child attempt to be accurate about jumping in the same spot repetitively.

▼ **CAUTION:** Take care that the child is jumping in a controlled fashion under supervision to prevent falling.

▶ Jumping Rope

Have the child jump unassisted for a period of 1 minute, followed by 1-minute rest. Increase in increments of 1 minute at a time. If the child is unable to jump unassisted, you can tie a long jump rope to a fence or doorknob and turn the rope for him.

▶ Running

Children love to run, especially when you make a game out of it.

Set up a course in the yard with cones or objects which the child can run through or around (an obstacle course of sorts). Use your imagination; you can make it as easy or difficult as you please.

It can be a simple running course laid out, or you can add little challenges like some small hurdles to jump over while running. Or make a relay race out of it by having the child carry and transfer little objects from one place to another. Get a stop watch and record his times; children love the challenge of beating their old scores or scores of friends or family members. For this activity the initial exercise should last at least 1 minute, and then slowly increase the duration. You can start off alternating running and walking and then build up to just running.

▶ *Jumping Jacks*

Show the child how to get in position with the feet together and arms at the side. Jump up and simultaneously raise the arms and spread the legs on the descent. Have the child perform 20 jumping jacks in a row, followed by a 15-second rest. Do a total of three sets. Once the child has mastered this, repeat with the child's eyes closed.

❖ BRAIN BALANCE PROFILE: *Nancy*

READING PROBLEM DISAPPEARS

Nancy was a sweet girl with a beautiful, easy smile. Everyone liked her, she had lots of friends, and teachers adored her. She was very personable and I could tell as soon as I met her that she could read people well. Her nonverbal skills were clearly excellent.

Her parents came to see me because she was struggling academically. Even though she was in fourth grade, she had difficulty reading. Despite coaching in school and at home, she simply could not sound out words. Now that she was getting older, her reading problem was starting to affect all her subjects. Her mother mentioned that it was getting harder and harder to motivate her—a problem, she assumed, that was the result of her reading problem. I noted that Nancy seemed to be a bit overweight and her mother agreed, adding that she seemed bloated much of the time.

Testing revealed that Nancy had a clear weakness of the left hemisphere. Her WIAT scores showed that her word reading and pseudoword decoding skills were much lower than her reading comprehension. Additional testing revealed that Nancy had good muscle tone but she displayed poor rhythm and timing. Plus, she struggled with fine motor skills, which was obvious by her terrible handwriting. Nancy was the classic dyslexic child.

The left hemisphere controls small muscles and small ideas. We use the left brain to decode the sound of a word. The left brain is all about details—the small picture. The right brain is in charge of big picture thinking. If the left brain is weak, a child cannot hear all the rapid changes in the sounds that make up words. She will be bad at phonics, mostly because the brain is processing sound and vision too slowly. This is what was wrong with Nancy. She was unable to match sound to the symbol (the letter), which is why she struggled reading words.

As is common in most children with dyslexia, Nancy was extremely perceptive in other areas. She could read people well and was very aware of her body in space—a well-grounded little girl. Her reading problem, however, was starting to interfere with her life.

We put Nancy on a left hemisphere program. Food tolerance testing confirmed that Nancy had a problem digesting milk products, which were the source of the bloating.

After three months, retesting revealed a dramatic increase in Nancy's left brain skills. She was now above grade level in all her academic skills. She also lost weight. After eliminating dairy from her diet, her bloating vanished.

The big reward, however, came in her report card at the end of the year. She went from getting C's and D's during first semester to straight A's in her last semester. Her symptoms of dyslexia were totally gone. Nancy now could read words as well as she could read people.

10

NEUROACADEMIC ASSESSMENT AND HOME ACTIVITIES

Aiming for a Better Grade

■

Joe's reading more fluently! His handwriting is looking
awesome and his attention span has definitely increased. Such
dramatic changes in such a small amount of time!
I'm so happy for him because I can tell
that he sees the positive changes, too.

—TEACHER'S NOTE TO JOE'S MOM

■

THE UNEVENNESS OF skills that is the hallmark of a child with Functional Disconnection Syndrome is most obvious when it comes to learning, homework, and grades.

A majority of children with learning disabilities, most notably those with ADHD, autism, and dyslexia, are actually quite bright, and have a great memory. They suffer from a knowledge gap, however, because their brain imbalance causes them to process information more slowly than normal. It's estimated that a child with ADHD is only paying attention in school 25 percent of the time. That's a lot of missed knowledge!

I am not the only person to recognize this unevenness of skills. For years, educators, psychologists, neuroscientists, and other professionals have noted that children in the spectrum of neurobehavioral and neuroacademic disorders struggle academically. The fact that a child can perform well, or even excel, at certain subjects and do poorly, or even fail, at others, has always been a conundrum. How can this be? The answer has always eluded them.

No one, until now, has recognized this as a problem caused by a brain imbalance. Children struggle academically because specific key functions in their brains that are used to perform specific academic tasks are underdeveloped. For example, a child can be a superior reader but struggle in class because his auditory system is out of balance. He can have perfect hearing but still not be able to process all of what a teacher is saying. Book learning is not a problem specifically, but learning in general is because he is not processing verbal instruction.

What we see is that academic strengths and weaknesses in different subjects can be broken down into left brain versus right brain ability. When you isolate the specific deficiency, you can find the cause, and then you can fix it.

I know many, many teachers and talk to them all the time. I really admire what they do, especially the veteran teachers who have been in the system for twenty or thirty years. They have played a key role in my investigation to find an answer to the unevenness of skills that is so apparent in the academic realm. I always gain a new insight every time I talk to a teacher.

The general tendency among educators when they are confronted with a child who excels at one thing and struggles at another is to encourage the child to build on the strength. When I explain to teachers why this is the worst thing they can do because it only makes an imbalance worse, it is like flipping the light switch. They totally get it.

If this is happening to your child in school, have it stopped. Take this book to your child's teacher and explain what you now know. Share the knowledge you are gaining. I do not know a teacher who would not appreciate this.

WHAT YOU CAN EXPECT

The exercises that you just read about in Chapter 9 are the basis of the Brain Balance Program and will, over time, make most, if not all, of the academic issues that your child is experiencing go away. I have seen children make amazing advances in their academic skills—many have even advanced multiple grade levels—in just twelve weeks on the Brain Balance Program.

Unfortunately, it is not going to fill the knowledge gap caused by your child's brain deficiency. You need to meet with your child's teacher or teachers and discuss this problem. If the gaps in your child's learning are not identified and replenished, your child may continue to struggle academically, even after the brain balance is corrected. To help you identify and correct your child's learning disabilities, this chapter offers:

■ Assessment checklists that will help you identify your child's academic problems as either left brain or right brain.
■ Instructions on how you can identify the specific academic skills that are challenging your child's potential, so that you can address them with teachers and tutors.
■ Academic exercises that will make all of this happen a little faster.

ACADEMIC ASSESSMENT CHECKLIST

Following is a list of thirty challenges that typically confront a child with either a left brain or a right brain deficiency. Consider them carefully and check off those that you feel describe your child. Discuss some of them with your child's teacher if you are not sure.

You should not expect to check off only left or only right brain issues. Nothing is ever that pure. But if your child has a brain imbalance, the results will definitely lean toward one side. Add this to the other evidence you have already collected in the other assessments.

▶ *Right Hemisphere Deficiency*

☐ Poor math reasoning (math word problems).
☐ Poor reading comprehension and pragmatic skills (misses the main idea or what a story character was thinking).
☐ Misses the big picture.
☐ Very analytical—processes ideas sequentially, step by step.
☐ Doesn't understand jokes.
☐ Very good at finding mistakes, such as spelling errors.
☐ Very literal.
☐ Speaks without reaching a conclusion.
☐ Early speech precociousness (talked well early).
☐ Was an early word reader.

- [ ] Has a fascination with letters and numbers.
- [ ] High IQ but with a noticeable disparity in skills.
- [ ] Interested in unusual topics.
- [ ] Learns in a rote (memorization) manner.
- [ ] Knows extraordinary amounts of specific facts about a subject, such as train schedules, TV schedules, baseball stats, world capitals.
- [ ] Excessively impatient.
- [ ] Displays poor voice inflection (speaks in a monotone with little or no expression).
- [ ] Poor sound levels in speech (speaks too loud or too soft).
- [ ] Poor nonverbal communication (can't read facial expressions or body posture).
- [ ] Speaks out loud regarding what he or she is thinking.
- [ ] Talks "in your face" (space invader).
- [ ] Good reader but does not enjoy reading.
- [ ] Thinks analytically. Makes logical deductions from information.
- [ ] Academic difficulties were picked up late because decoding and spelling were very strong.
- [ ] Likes to make lists and plan.
- [ ] Follows rules without questioning them.
- [ ] Easily memorizes spelling and mathematical formulas.
- [ ] Enjoys observing rather than participating.
- [ ] More likely to read an instruction manual before trying something new.
- [ ] Math was the first subject that was problematic.

Total _____

▶ Left Hemisphere Deficiency

- [ ] Very good at big picture skills.
- [ ] Intuitive thinker—led by feelings.
- [ ] Good at abstract "free" association.
- [ ] Poor analytical skills (has difficulty breaking things into smaller parts).
- [ ] Inquisitive about what others are doing or why rules exist.
- [ ] Difficulty with prioritizing.

☐ Unlikely to read instruction manual before trying something new.

☐ Naturally creative, but needs to apply self to develop potential.

☐ Would rather do than observe.

☐ Misreads or omits common small words.

☐ Had difficulty naming colors, objects, and letters as a small child.

☐ Needs to hear or see concepts many times in order to learn them.

☐ Is exhibiting downward scores in achievement tests and/or school performance.

☐ Schoolwork is inconsistent.

☐ Was late in learning to talk.

☐ Has difficulty pronouncing words (poor with phonics).

☐ Had difficulty learning the alphabet, nursery rhymes, or songs as a small child.

☐ Acts before thinking.

☐ Makes careless mistakes.

☐ Reads slowly. Tends to misread, omit, or repeat words.

☐ Sometimes writes letters backward.

☐ Poor at math operations—has difficulty counting or calculating, such as long division.

☐ Had above-average number of ear infections.

☐ Has a poor memory for facts and figures.

☐ Has poor academic ability.

☐ Performs poorly on verbal tests.

☐ Needs to be told something several times.

☐ Spells poorly.

☐ Poor test performer—doesn't read directions well and misinterprets questions.

☐ Has poor memorization skills.

Total _____

ACADEMIC MILESTONES ASSESSMENT

Because signs of a brain deficiency often show up early—in some children even before they are born—many clues can be found when looking back.

These milestones pertain exclusively to language and verbal development. Read through them and recall the age at which your child achieved these specific skills. You don't have to write anything down or keep a tally. It is just one more assessment that will help you determine if your child has FDS and if it is due to a left or a right brain delay.

At the age of six months, a child should be:

Making many different sounds, including laughing, gurgling, and cooing.

Reacting to tone of voice, especially if loud or angry.

Turning in the direction of new sounds, such as toys that rattle and squeak or a song being sung.

Babbling to get attention, using sounds that include *p*, *b*, and *in*.

Smiling when spoken to.

Indicating a need for something through sound or gesture.

At eight months, a child should be:

Responding to his or her name.

Saying at least four or more different, distinct sounds.

Using syllables such as *da*, *ba*, and *ka*.

Listening to his or her own voice and others' voices.

Trying to imitate some sounds.

Responding to the word "no."

Participating in games such as peekaboo.

At ten months, a child should be:

Making utterances that sound like *mama* or *dada*, but not necessarily labeled to the person.

Making noncrying sounds to attract attention, such as squealing or raising the voice.

Connecting syllables that sound like real speech, including both long and short groups of sounds.

Repeating certain syllables or sequences of sounds over and over.

At one year, a child should be:

Recognizing her name and turning to look when she hears her
name.

Saying "mama" and "dada" and maybe two or three additional
words.

Imitating familiar words and animal sounds.

Understanding simple commands and instructions, such as
"come here."

Able to wave and understand "bye-bye."

Able to make appropriate eye contact and show affection for
familiar people.

Responding to sounds such as the doorbell ringing or the dog
barking.

Understanding that words are symbols for objects.

Understanding the meaning of the word "no," even if she doesn't
agree.

At eighteen months, a child should be:

Using at least five to ten words, including names of people and
familiar things.

Using some words to express wants or needs, such as "more."

Pointing and gesturing to a desired object.

Starting to combine two words, such as "all gone."

Pointing to familiar body parts.

Recognizing pictures of familiar things and people.

Getting familiar objects upon request, even if in another room.

Getting more accurate at imitating sounds and words.

Responding when his or her name is called.

Humming or singing simple tunes.

Listening and responding to quiet speech.

At age two, a child should:

Use two- to three-word "sentences," such as "No want" and "No
go."

Have a vocabulary of approximately 200 to 300 words and use
about 150 regularly.

Show affection for familiar people.

Express simple desires or needs for familiar things or actions
    through speaking rather than pointing.
Refer to self by name rather than "me" or "I."
Ask "why" questions, such as "What that?" and "Where kitty?"
Understand simple questions and commands.
Name familiar pictures.

At two and a half years, a child should:

Know the names of family members and others.
Have a 400-word vocabulary and be able to name familiar objects
    and pictures.
Say his or her first name and hold up fingers to show his or her age.
Say "no," though it may mean "yes."
Refer to self as "me" rather than by name.
Answer "where" questions.
Use short sentences regularly, such as "Me do it."
Use past tense and plurals, although not always correctly.
Be talking to other children and adults.
Know how to match at least three colors.
Know the difference between big and little.

At age three years, a child should:

Speak and be understood by strangers, even though many articu-
    lation errors may persist.
Have a vocabulary of nearly 1,000 words.
Name at least one color and be able to match all primary colors.
Know concepts such as night and day, boy and girl, big and little,
    in and out.
Follow two-step requests, such as "Get the toy and put it in the box."
Sing familiar songs.
Talk a lot (to self and others).

At age four, a child should:

Have a vocabulary of 1,500 words.
Use four- to five-word sentences.

Begin to use more complex sentences.

Use plurals, contractions, and past tense.

Ask many questions, including "why?"

Understand simple "who," "what," and "where" questions.

Follow commands and directions, even if the target object is not present.

Identify some basic shapes, such as circle and square.

Identify primary colors.

Talk about concepts in the abstract and imaginary conditions, such as "I hope Santa brings me a scooter."

Begin to copy patterns, such as lines and circles on a page.

Pay attention to a short story and may be able to answer questions about it.

Hear and understand most of what is said at home and in preschool.

Relate incidents that happened in school or at home.

At age five, a child should:

Have a 2,000-word vocabulary.

Speak in five- to six-word sentences.

Use different types of sentences, including complex ones that describe cause and effect or temporal relations, such as "I'll get in trouble if I hit Jimmy" or "I can have a cookie after I eat my lunch."

Use past, present, and future tenses.

Count to 10, including counting objects.

Understand what objects are used for and made of.

Know spatial relationships, such as behind, far, near, and on top of.

Comprehend the concept of opposites, such as hard/soft, long/short.

Ask questions for the purpose of gaining new information.

Know right and left on self, but not necessarily on others.

Express feelings, dreams, wishes, and other abstract thoughts.

Copy basic capital letters when shown an example.

Can draw rudimentary pictures.

Perhaps be able to write his name.

Although some children may be able to spell or read by age five, these skills are not the norm.

COMMON SIGNS OF LEARNING DISABILITIES

Again, think back and see if you recognize any of these traits as
they pertained to your child.

▶ *Preschool*

Does not speak as much as most of the other children.
Has trouble with pronunciation.
Has slow vocabulary growth.
Is often unable to find the right word when communicating.
Is not very good at rhyming words.
Has trouble learning numbers, alphabet, days of the week, colors,
shapes.
Is extremely restless and easily distracted.
Has trouble interacting with peers.
Has difficulty following directions or routines.
Has slow development of fine motor skills.

▶ *Kindergarten Through Grade 4*

Is slow to learn the connection between letters and sounds.
Confuses basic words, such as *run*, *eat*, and *want*.
Makes consistent reading and spelling errors, including letter
reversals (*b/d*), inversions (*m/w*), transpositions (*felt/left*), and
substitutions (*house/home*).
Transposes number sequences and confuses arithmetic signs
(+, -, x, /, =).
Is slow to remember facts.
Is slow to learn new skills and relies heavily on memorization.
Is impulsive.
Has difficulty planning.
Has an unstable pencil grip.
Has trouble learning about time.
Has poor coordination.
Is unaware of physical surroundings.
Is prone to accidents.

▶ *Grades 5 Through 8*

Reverses letter sequences (*soiled/solid, left/felt*).

Is slow to learn prefixes, suffixes, root words, and other spelling strategies.

Avoids reading aloud.

Has trouble with word problems.

Has difficulty with handwriting.

Has awkward, fistlike, or tight pencil grip.

Avoids writing assignments.

Has slow or poor recall of facts.

Has difficulty making friends.

Has trouble understanding body language and facial expressions.

▶ *Grades 9 Through 12*

Is a poor speller and frequently spells the same word differently in a single piece of writing.

Avoids reading and writing tasks.

Has trouble summarizing.

Has trouble answering open-ended test questions.

Has weak memory skills.

Has difficulty adjusting to new settings.

Performs tasks slowly.

Has a poor grasp of abstract concepts.

Either pays too little attention to details or focuses on them too much.

Misreads information.

WHAT A REPORT CARD CAN TELL YOU

There is a lot you can learn about your child's brain development from his or her report card. But it is not enough just to read the marks and see what subjects are problematic. You need to find out what is *behind* the marks. The reason? There are almost no subjects that are purely left or right brain. Hemispheric skill sets come into play in all of them—another obvious explanation as to why the brain needs to be functioning as a whole.

▶ *Reading Early Reports*

When it comes to report cards, here is an important tip, especially when it comes to preschool and kindergarten: They tend to be somewhat subjective. They are often slanted to the viewpoint of the teacher. Nevertheless, there is plenty that you can read into them. When you look at the report card, ask yourself these questions:

- Is your child learning the basic foundational skills well—shapes, colors, letters, numbers, and so forth? If not, this is usually an early sign of a left brain deficit.
- Is the report card pointing out problems in the primary areas that are foundational to other academic skills, or are most of the teacher's comments about behavior or attitude—not applying himself and the like? Behavioral problems usually signify a right hemisphere delay whereas academic problems usually signify a left hemisphere delay.
- Does your child seem to be learning basic skills adequately, but there is criticism about attention span and being disruptive in class? This is usually specific to a right brain delay.

▶ *Other Grades*

As children progress into elementary and later grades, report cards are based more on test grades, classroom participation, and homework. This becomes more objective. But again, reading a grade is not enough of an answer. For one, there are almost as many different types of report cards as there are states in the nation.

When children come to our centers, we always look at their report cards, but we also administer our own test to come up with a more complete and objective report card.

We use a standardized test that measures academic achievement. There are many different kinds of tests that school districts can use, but the most common are the Wechsler Individual Achievement Test II, known simply as the WIAT II, and the Woodcock Johnston III. I have found the WIAT to be the better of the two.

Keep in mind, however, that there is almost no one subject that is purely left brain or right brain. For instance, reading is a major skill subject. Many teachers and parents think the child can either read well or not read well. But what they often discover from a standardized test is that certain reading skills are good and others are poor. From a traditional perspective, this doesn't make any sense and there hasn't been a satisfactory explanation for it. However, what we do makes sense, because we analyze the skill sets within the test by hemispheric brain function. Grading deficits in children with FDS clearly lean either left or right.

Here I am showing you how academic tests are designed and how we analyze them—and you can, too—for skill value. As a parent, you have the right to review your child's test scores and your request to do so should be granted. You will gain amazing insight when you read the results the way we do in Brain Balance. This can also be very helpful if you are using a private tutor, as it will show what to focus on.

READING THE GRADE THE BRAIN BALANCE WAY

The WIAT test is broken into nine primary subject areas, which are further broken into subsets. We have taken most of these subject areas and subsets and broken them into left brain and right brain skill sets. Use the information below to do your own analysis of your child's academic tests. Since most tests use a format similar to the WIAT's, you should be able to apply this information to the standardized academic test used in your school district. Each major subject area is further broken down to several subsets in the error analysis section of the WIAT. If you get your child's report, make sure you also get the error analysis, and look at those scores. Ask a professional to help you if you need assistance to understand the scoring. Compare the results of each section of the error analysis to the guide we have included below to clearly see if your child has a right brain or a left brain delay.

▶ 1. Word Reading

This measures how well your child can read words by sounding out letters, what in academia is known as phonological awareness and decoding. In general, it is a left brain skill. It tests:

Letter identification
Phonological awareness

Alphabet (letter-sound knowledge)
Accuracy of word recognition
Automaticity of word recognition

Letter identification. A small picture detail and therefore a left brain skill. Recognition has much to do with memory, and memory for detail is also a left brain skill. A letter is easier to identify if a child can link it to a particular sound. In dyslexia, reversal and transposition of letters are common—the letters are hard to remember because of a problem with phonological awareness.

Phonological awareness. Also a left brain skill. These are the sounds that make up words and the child has to hear them all. This ability requires a good auditory system because the child needs to process the individual sounds very quickly. However, a child won't be able to hear all the sounds if the auditory circuits in the left brain are too slow.

Alphabet. A left brain skill because letters are symbols and are dependent on overall processing speed.

Accuracy of word recognition. A left brain skill. Remembering and recognizing words are basically the same process as letter recognition; you can't effectively have one without the other.

Automaticity of word recognition. Once the brain learns something, the information is supposed to become automated. To remember something, the brain has to be repeatedly exposed to it. The left brain is the conscious learning center. If a child can't read a word, it won't store the information for the memory to retrieve.

Conclusion: Word reading as a subject is clearly a left brain skill.

▶ 2. Reading Comprehension

This measures the ability to read and understand the meaning of written passages. Questions are geared to measure:

Literal comprehension
Inferential comprehension
Lexical comprehension
Reading rate
Oral reading accuracy

Oral reading fluency
Oral reading comprehension
Word recognition in context
Main idea

Reading comprehension, in general, is a right brain skill. However, a child needs to be able to use both sides of the brain to do it well. Reading comprehension is the single most common problem in children with a right brain deficit. Most parents believe that if their child can recite a story and remember the details, then he understands what he is reading. Not necessarily. Remembering details is small picture thinking (left brain) but comprehension is big picture thinking (right brain). The error analysis will make the difference clearer.

Literal comprehension. Most children with a right brain deficiency are very literal—they take the meaning of a word for exactly what it is. They don't understand that a single word can mean more than one thing. Alternate meanings are often dependent on nonverbal clues. For example, changing the inflection of your voice to make a declarative sentence into a question can be missed in a child with a right brain problem. Understanding the literal meaning is small detail, so it is a left brain skill.

Inferential comprehension. This is the exact opposite of literal comprehension, and it is a right brain skill. It is what makes reading fun. "To infer" means to be able to figure out something that is not explicitly said. This is inherent in reading comprehension.

When you are reading with your child, you should ask questions about the story. *Why did the witch say that to Snow White?*

Lexical comprehension. Understanding the meanings of words is primarily a right brain skill, although it has features of both sides. As detail, it seems to be left brain, but it is really more right brain because to really understand the meaning of the word, you must understand its context.

Reading rate. As a skill, it is primarily left brain. To do it well depends on several factors, including coordination of eye movements, which happens in the right brain. Rapidly sequential activities are a left brain skill.

Oral reading accuracy. A left brain skill very much like word recognition.

Oral reading fluency. Speed and fluency, whether reading to oneself or aloud, is a left brain skill.

Oral reading comprehension. Primarily right brain because it is big picture thinking. However, it also involves recalling details, which is left brain.

Word recognition in context. The left brain is about content (details, facts); the right is about context (meaning, big picture).

Main idea. The main idea is the big picture, so it is a right brain skill. The child needs to be able to step back and put all the pieces together to figure out the bigger meaning, what is called global processing. Some children can't do this because they get stuck in the detail.

Conclusion: Out of the nine subsets that comprise reading comprehension, four require left brain skills and five require right brain skills. So, if reading comprehension is a problem, you need to look into what aspects of the skill are causing the problem. But generally, reading comprehension is considered a right brain skill.

▶ 3. Pseudoword Decoding

This measures the ability to apply the skills of sounding out words. Subsets include:

Phonological decoding
Accuracy of word attack

These are both left brain skills. To test these skills, WIAT uses pseudowords—fake words. This is because children may already be familiar with some words from hearing them. This ability is dependent mostly on auditory processing in the left brain. We have discovered that a problem with this ability automatically corrects itself through the Brain Balance Program. This is where auditory exercises come into play.

Conclusion: Pseudoword decoding is clearly left brain.

▶ 4. Numerical Operations

This evaluates a child's ability to identify and write numbers and solve simple equations involving all main math operations. Subsets are:

Counting
One-to-one correspondence
Numerical identification and writing

Calculation

Fractions, decimals, algebra

Counting. This basic math function is linear and logical, a small picture skill and definitely left brain.

One-to-one correspondence. Details, left brain.

Numerical identification and writing. Like writing and word recognition, very left brain.

Calculation. This consists of the basic math operations, so it is a left brain skill.

Fractions, decimals, algebra. The left brain is good at figuring out how new information shares something in common with other, similar data that is already known. It is especially good at step-by-step algebra.

Conclusion: Like word reading, it is primarily a left brain skill.

▧ Your Typical Math Wizard ▧

MATHEMATICAL talent is a fascinating interest to neuropsychologists. It is defined as a high level of math reasoning ability at an early age. There are several unique features about extremely gifted math students:

They are more likely to be male than female.

Fifty percent are either left-handed or ambidextrous.

More than fifty percent have allergies (more than twice the rate of the general population).

It is also a sign of a brain imbalance. It is a sign of increased right brain function and decreased left brain ability. ▪

▶ *5. Math Reasoning*

This evaluates conceptual knowledge, the ability to reason mathematically by interpreting graphs, solving word problems, and identifying patterns. Math reasoning uses right brain spatial skills and mental rotation skills. Males, who are more right brain, are generally better at higher-level math concepts, especially beyond the fifth grade and into high school. Boys statistically score higher than girls on the math section of the SAT. Studies show, however, that girls generally do better than boys at basic math skills.

Conceptual knowledge, in general, is a big picture, abstract type of skill—very right brain. This requires reasoning skills that even in math are more right brain.

Multistep problem solving
Money, time, and measurement
Geometry
Reading and interpreting charts and graphs
Statistics and probability
Estimation
Identifying patterns

Multistep problem solving. Following step-by-step instructions is a sequential skill—left brain.

Money, time, and measurement. Understanding the relationship between space and time is called a visuospatial math skill, the kind credited for Einstein's genius. Formulating the theory of relativity is probably the biggest big picture concept ever.

Geometry. The ability to picture things in three dimensions and mentally rotate objects in space is very spatial and a right brain ability. This ability takes place in the right orbital frontal cortex, which is the first area to develop in males.

Reading and interpreting charts and graphs. Details, details—reading numbers and looking at graphs—all very left brain. Children diagnosed with Asperger's are particularly skilled in this area.

Statistics and probability. This skill involves following precise rules. It is the definition of logic. It is a pattern recognition skill that resides in the left brain.

Estimation. This involves intuitive and abstract thinking—both right brain.

Identifying patterns. This is the skill that is used to play computer games—a left brain skill.

Conclusion: As with reading comprehension, math reasoning involves both sides of the brain. This is why you can't draw a conclusion based on math reasoning in general. You have to look deeper. But in general math reasoning is a right brain skill.

▶ *6. Spelling*

This evaluates a child's ability to remember letters and words. Subsets include:

Alphabet principle
Written spelling of regular and irregular words
Written spelling of homonyms

Conclusion: Generally, spelling is a left brain skill.

▶ *7. Written Expression*

This measures a child's ability to demonstrate written word fluency, generate sentences, and form a sentence or paragraph. Subsets include:

Timed alphabet writing
Written word fluency
Sentence combining
Sentence generation
Written response to verbal and visual clues
Descriptive writing
Writing fluency

Timed alphabet writing. This requires fine motor skills and the ability to sequentially recall letters, both left brain skills.

Written word fluency. Fluency is language and therefore also a left brain function.

Sentence combining. Putting sentences together requires the ability to derive meaning and convey a concept. The left brain can form a sentence but putting them together in a cohesive paragraph requires big picture thinking. So this is largely a right brain skill.

Sentence generation. This is the ability to write creatively, a right brain skill.

Written response to verbal and visual clues. This is all about imagination and intuitive thinking. It requires the ability to intuit what the person giving the clues is thinking. It brings nonverbal skills into play, which is right brain.

Descriptive writing. This is evaluated for organization, vocabulary, the ability to develop a theme, and the basic mechanics of writing. When writing something that someone else is going to read, the writer has to be able to think like the reader. This is a right brain skill.

Writing fluency. This is measured by word count, a left brain skill.

Conclusion: This subject area needs to be examined carefully because it requires both left and right brain skills. Right brain functions, however, are generally more important to achieve a satisfactory grade in written expression. Being able to really understand what the reader will be thinking and feeling is what written expression is all about. It requires written thought that taps into emotions and feelings. Vocabulary and the basic function of writing itself are left brain requirements.

▶ 8. Listening Comprehension

This measures a child's ability to listen for detail. This takes a variety of skills that are both left and right brain. Subsets are:

Expressive vocabulary
Listening-inferential comprehension

Expressive vocabulary. Speech resides in the left brain and is therefore a left brain function.

Listening-inferential comprehension. The ability to listen and infer requires intuitive thinking and nonverbal skills. These are right brain skills.

Conclusion: Being successful in listening comprehension involves both left and right brain skills. Generally this can be looked at as more of a right brain skill.

▶ 9. Oral Expression

This measures a child's ability to generate stories and get direction from visual and verbal cues. It would seem that this would be a left brain function, but it is not that clear-cut. Subsets include:

Word fluency (oral)
Auditory short-term recall for contextual information
Story generation
Giving directions
Explaining steps in sequential task
Sequentially following tasks

Word fluency. From everything you've read so far, this is obviously a left brain skill.

Auditory short-term recall for contextual information. This means using short-term memory, which requires the ability to pay attention. This is a right brain skill. It also requires big picture thinking, also a right brain skill.

Story generation. This requires imagination and an awareness of the person listening or reading, a right brain function.

Giving directions. Obviously, this requires spatial knowledge, a right hemisphere ability. (By the way, most men tend to be right-brained, which is why they are pretty good at directions. Being right-brained also makes them nonverbal, which is why when they get lost, they try to avoid asking for directions!)

Explaining steps in sequential tasks. Anything that is sequential and involves step-by-step tasks is left brain.

Sequentially following steps. This is the kind of skill in which left brainers excel.

Conclusion: I have seen children with both left and right brain delays do poorly on this aspect of the test. As a result of the Brain Balance Program, I have also seen big gains in this area—as much as ten grade levels. The biggest gains are seen in kids with a right brain delay.

IMPROVING COGNITIVE SKILLS

Reading the results of a WIAT test in the manner I just described will clearly show you the deficits in your child's learning ability. These deficits are what are really behind your child's poor grades. To correct them requires giving your child frequent drills in his or her specific areas of weakness. It is beyond the scope of this book to give drills for all the skills at all the grade levels. However, there are many workbooks available specifically designed to help you achieve this. Many of them are teacher resource books—nontextbooks—and can be found in bookstores and on the Internet. These books are filled with drills targeted to specific subjects at specific grade levels. The following are examples of some of these drills. They are aimed at a fourth grade level unless otherwise specified.

▶ Literal Comprehension Exercise

Use any book at your child's reading level to do this exercise. The point is to find out if your child can comprehend the main idea of a passage. For example:

Sit quietly with your child so he can concentrate and read him a passage from a book or article such as this one: "Did you know that just a small part of all the salt in the world is put into food to make the food taste better? There are hundreds of other uses for salt, though. In the United States more salt is used for melting snow and ice on roads than for any other purpose." Then give your child a multiple-choice question such as:

The story's main theme is:
- A. Two uses of salt
- B. How to melt snow
- C. How to chop ice

▶ Inferential Comprehension Exercise

This exercise tests your child's ability to use vague clues in a story to find out what is really being said—that is, to "read between the lines." It is like a guessing game, and you can make this fun. For example:

Little Tommy saw a crowd of children on the playground. He went over to see what the kids were doing. In the middle of the crowd a mother was painting a picture of her child. Tommy looked at the picture and said, "I wish she would paint my picture." Which of the following is true? Which is false? Which is an inference?

- A. No one was watching the mother paint.
- B. The mother was painting on the playground.
- C. Tommy thought the woman was a good artist.

▶ *Oral Reading Comprehension Exercise*

Before children learn how to effectively read silently, they need to master the ability to read and comprehend aloud. It is called "getting the main idea." Use exercises like this to test and improve your child's ability in this area. Describe a story such as the following:

A baby oyster is the size of a pinpoint. It takes a month for it to grow to the size of a pea. In one year it is as big as a quarter. From then on, the oyster grows about an inch a year for three or four years.
    The story tells mainly:

A. How fast oysters grow.
B. What oysters like to eat.
C. Why oysters grow so fast.

Here is another example:

Hundreds of years ago, lead pencils were actually made of lead. Today they are made of graphite. Graphite makes a much darker mark than lead. It lasts a long time, too. A pencil has enough graphite in it to draw a line thirty-two miles long.
    The main idea of this story is:

A. How pencils were invented.
B. Why pencils are made of graphite.
C. Who discovered graphite.

▶ *Pseudoword Decoding Exercise*

Test your child's ability to sound out words by having him read a list of nonsense pseudowords aloud. Make up your own words. Such as:

1. nat
2. lut
3. tunk
4. fing

• • •

▶ *One-to-One Correspondence Exercise*

Illustrate the relationship between verbal language and the written word by pointing to a word and having the child say it aloud. This is considered an early form of one-to-one correspondence.

▶ *Numerical Identification and Identifying Exercise*

Younger children need to be able to identify numbers and letters and then be able to verbally discuss them. Pointing to numbers that are not in order and asking a child to identify them is an example of numerical identification.

▶ *Calculation Exercise*

This includes basic addition, subtraction, multiplication, and division. Examples would be:

A. $6 + 8 = $ _____
B. $10 - 5 = $ _____
C. $9 \times 4 = $ _____
D. $15 / 3 = $ _____

▶ *Math Reasoning Exercise*

This is the ability to solve word problems. For example:

Sue likes to collect seashells. On Friday she had 23 shells in her collection. On Saturday she went back to the beach and collected 8 more shells. Sue then went to the store and bought 19 more shells for $5.50. At a nearby garage sale she purchased 6 more shells. At the end of the day how many shells did Sue have in her collection?

▶ *Multistep Problem Solving Exercise*

Here is an example of a fifth-grade multistep problem:

Brad and Jill have 28 coins. Jill and Bill have 35 coins. Brad and Bill have 21 coins. How many coins does Brad have?

▶ *Listening Comprehension Exercise*

This tests the ability to listen carefully and comprehend what is being read. This can be measured by the child's answers to questions that are directly related to the passage read. For example:

When is a bear not a bear? Does that sound like a riddle with a tricky answer? It isn't! A bear is not a bear when it is a koala. The koala is a small animal of Australia. Mother koalas have a pouch, like that of a kangaroo or an opossum.
A koala is a small animal of:

A. Australia
B. China
C. America

COGNITIVE SKILLS EXERCISES

Most developmental delays in both right and left hemispheres involve the frontal lobes, the large area of the brain responsible for the skills required in higher-level learning and thinking. It involves the ability to focus, pay attention, concentrate without getting distracted, and shift from one thought or idea to another. The following exercises are designed to refine these skills. They are not part of the formal Brain Balance Program so you can do them at will. You can also use them as another measure of progress as you move through the program. They are a lot of fun. Both parents and children enjoy them.

▶ *Contrasting Programs*

Sit facing your child. Hold up one hand and instruct your child as follows: *Hold up one hand opposite mine. As soon as I raise one finger, you raise two fingers. When I put my finger down, you put yours down. Whenever I raise two fingers, you raise only one finger. Respond as quickly as possible, and put your finger down each time as soon as you have responded.* Use a quasirandom pattern, such as 1, 1, 1, 2, 1, 2, 2, 1, 1, 2. Do this test a total of ten times and record how often the child failed to follow.

It is normal to make one or two errors in each set. If your child makes more, you should see improvement fairly quickly as you move through the program.

▶ Go No-Go

After completing the contrasting programs test, instruct the child: *Now I am going to change the rules. When I hold up one finger, you still hold up two, but now when I hold up two fingers, you don't hold up any.* Begin with the sequence, 1, 1, 1, 1, 2, and continue using a quasirandom pattern. Do this test a total of ten times and record how often the child failed to follow.

Again, it is normal to make one or two errors in each set. If your child makes more, you should see improvement fairly quickly as you move through the program.

▶ Eye Movement (Antisaccade) Exercise

Saccade refers to rapid eye movements. This exercise is exactly the same as the Fast-Eye Tracking exercises you did in Chapter 9 (review this before starting) though the instructions are different. Instead of looking at a wiggling finger, the child will look at the opposite finger. The natural impulse is to look at the moving finger. The child has to inhibit the impulse to look at the moving finger and do the opposite.

Stand face-to-face with your child. Hold up both of your hands so one is in the visual field of each of your child's eyes. Ask your child to look you in the eye. Tell him that when you wiggle a finger of one hand, he should look at the opposite hand. Do this a total of ten times, using a quasirandom sequence with each round. But try to use one hand more than the other. If the child has a right brain deficit, wiggle your right hand more so that the child will look left, which will stimulate the right brain. For the left brain, favor your right finger more than the left.

▶ Word Fluency Exercise

Ask your child to recite as many words as possible that begin with a specific letter within a minute. She cannot use proper nouns (names, places) or repeat variations of a word, such as *great, greater, greatest*. Use a stop watch or the second hand of your watch to time her. Give the signal "go" to begin. Standard letters to use are A, F, and S. If she stops before the minute is up, give her one brief reminder to keep going but no more. Count the number of words she says but subtract words that are not allowed to get your true total.

Typically, a child can find twelve words beginning with each letter.

▶ *Visual Processing Skill*

These exercises test both detail and big picture skills. Have your child look at each of the following and ask him what he sees. This will activate one side of the brain and inhibit the other.

```
V
V
V
V
V  V  V  V  V  V  V  V
```

If the child sees a V, he is using his left brain; if he sees an L, he is using his right brain. You can make up a bunch of letters like this one and do the test several times a week. But if you tell him to focus on only the small letter or the big letter, you can activate one side of the brain more specifically.

■ **Academic Problem or Behavior Problem?** ■

YOU may think your child has one or the other, but your child really has both—or at least he will, unless you correct it first.

The more common right brain deficiency, such as we see with ADHD and autism, usually starts as a behavior problem, so it is usually discovered early on. The less common left brain deficit, such as dyslexia, usually starts out as an academic problem, so it often isn't "caught" until after a child enters school.

The two, however, are closely intertwined. Academic struggles usually breed behavior problems and behavior problems generally cause academic troubles. This usually becomes apparent around the fourth grade when subject matter starts to get more difficult.

It is important that a corrective program begin as soon as a problem is detected. A brain imbalance gets more pronounced the longer it exists, making the road to recovery more difficult. However, recovery can take place at any age. It is never too late.   ▪

BRAIN BALANCE PROFILE: *Davis*

FROM SPECIAL ED TO GIFTED PROGRAM

Davis was almost ten and in the fifth grade when his mother brought him to our Brain Balance Center. Davis had been diagnosed with ADHD three years earlier and he also suffered from severe headaches.

Although his intelligence was quite obvious, his mother said he was placed in a special education class for most of his time in school because he couldn't pay attention and he was easily distracted. I could see that this was very distressing to her. The doctor who diagnosed his ADHD put him on two powerful antiseizure medications, Depakote and Neurontin. His parents had tried various programs, such as behavioral modification and private tutors, to help control the ADHD but they didn't help. Now his headaches were getting worse and more frequent. His parents' main concern when they came to see me was to get rid of his headaches and get him off the medication.

Our Brain Balance testing process found that Davis had a very clear neurological imbalance and he fit the profile of a child with a right hemisphere delay—typical for a child with ADHD. Davis also had physical signs of the imbalance. He had poor spatial awareness— and poor coordination between the two sides of his body. He also had a pronounced right-sided head tilt, which we strongly suspected was the cause of his headaches.

Academically, he had the unevenness of skills so typical of children with Functional Disconnection Syndrome and the typical learning and behavior patterns we see with boys who are diagnosed with ADHD.

His attention deficit was readily obvious when we put him through the Wechsler Individual Achievement Test (WIAT), the gold standard for evaluating academic achievement. Despite this disability and the fact that he was in a special education class, Davis nevertheless tested near the ninth-grade level in most left brain subjects. On right brain subjects, he tested at second-, third-, and fifth-grade levels.

We put Davis on a program that included right hemisphere exercises. We explained to his mother that the headaches were a manifestation of the head tilt that was caused by the brain imbalance. We explained that fixing the imbalance would cure all Davis's problems, including his ADHD.

We worked with Davis at our center, and his mother dutifully worked on his home assignments. The reduction in the frequency and severity of the headaches alone delighted his mother because this was her goal to begin with. So you can imagine the thrill she was in for when, three months from day one, we once again put him through WIAT testing and found a marked improvement. On left brain subjects he stayed the same, which was exactly what we wanted to happen. On right brain subjects, his score shot up 5.8 years in reading comprehension, 8 years in math reasoning, 3.4 years in written expression, and 7 years in listening comprehension—an average increase of 6.5 years in eight subjects. Also, Davis's headaches all but disappeared, and his doctor took him off the medication. Retesting also confirmed he no longer fit the diagnostic criteria for ADHD. The real bonus, however, came a month after he ended our program when he was taken out of special ed and placed immediately into a gifted program.

That was three years ago. I saw Davis's mom recently and she told me that, on occasion, he still gets the same old headaches but he tolerates them well and doesn't need medication. And, she mentioned proudly, "Davis has been on the honor roll every semester since he left your program."

11

WHAT SHOULD I FEED MY CHILD?

Brain Balance Nutrition Plan

■

Sometimes hope takes the shape of a six-year-old boy
who inhaled the smell of freshly baked chocolate chip cookies
for the first time.

—MARYBETH G.

■

PASTA, PIZZA, BAGELS, milk, cereal, macaroni and cheese. Are these among your child's favorite food groups? If not all of them, it's a good bet that at least some of these foods fit into your child's menu several times a week, if not almost daily.

Kids have been fussy eaters since, well, maybe not the beginning of all time but at least since the beginning of modern time when provisions became plentiful and man created fast-food chains and the scourge known as trans fat.

It is hardly a secret these days that the typical American diet is taking its toll on the health of our children (as well as adults) in terms of the rising rate of obesity and the earlier onset of serious but avoidable health threats, such as heart disease and diabetes. There hasn't been enough emphasis, however, on how poor eating habits are jeopardizing the development of a healthy brain.

The brain's primary fuels are oxygen and glucose, which are manufactured from nutrients in our food supply. A brain that has plenty of stimulation but too little fuel will not be able to take advantage of that stimulation.

Without fuel, the brain can't make new proteins to build new branches or make and repair cells that produce energy. Without fuel, brain cells will fatigue, get damaged, and die. Stimulation without fuel, or fuel without stimulation, does not work.

Poor nutrition is a big threat to the development of a healthy brain because children do not eat properly. Many children are fussy eaters and exasperated parents will let kids eat anything they want just so they eat.

A study published in the *Journal of Pediatrics* paints a sorry portrait of the nutritional health of American children. According to the report:

Only 1 percent of young people between the ages of two and nineteen eat a healthy diet.

On average, the same age group gets 40 percent of daily caloric intake in the form of fat, most of it dangerous saturated fat.

The National Academy of Sciences estimates that 12 million children get fewer nutrients than they need every day for optimum health. Yet, kids today are too fat, which means that they are eating too many calories. This in itself is proof that there is something very wrong with the way parents are feeding their children.

WHAT KIDS SHOULD BE EATING

There is nothing special about the kinds of food that are healthy for the brain. They are the exact same foods that children need for optimum overall health. Children should be getting *per day*:

6 to 11 servings of grains
3 to 5 servings of vegetables
2 to 4 servings of fruit
2 to 3 servings of dairy products
5 to 7 ounces of meat

Kids today are not getting anywhere near these levels of nutrients. One study of more than 3,300 children between the ages of two and nineteen found that less than 1 percent of children are getting sufficient amounts of fruits, vegetables, grains, and other foods that supply the nutrients essential to healthy brain and body growth.

This should come as no big surprise to parents who struggle daily to fill their child's plate with adequate nutrition. Many kids are fussy eaters but kids with FDS are exceptionally finicky. This causes an additional dilemma for you because children with FDS have compromises in the body that make absorption of nutrients difficult. The problems include:

An underdeveloped digestive system, which may cause a
   "leaking gut."
Reduced ability to secrete acids that chemically break down food.
Reduced muscle contractions (peristalsis) which mechanically
   break down food.
Reduced ability to absorb nutrients from food.
Decreased blood circulation in the intestines and stomach lining.

So even if a child with FDS eats a healthy well-balanced diet every day, chances are he or she will still end up nutritionally deficient.

GETTING TO THE SOURCE OF THE PROBLEM

There are two nutritional components that you need to address in order to resolve your child's brain imbalance. One is discovering and eliminating sensitive foods that exacerbate Functional Disconnection Syndrome and the other is restoring depleted vitamin stores.

A child with FDS has special nutritional challenges that are not all that easy to pinpoint. However, this chapter offers the guidance that should enable you to do both quite handily on your own.

If you want to enlist professional help, I recommend that you see a nutritionist who has expertise in childhood nutrition and preferably one who has treated children with autism, ADHD, or any of the other neurological disorders discussed in this book.

Take this book with you when you make your appointment. It is imperative that the nutritionist understands the underlying causes of your child's brain imbalance and its nutritional repercussions.

You need to start making these important nutritional changes at the same time you begin the Brain Balance exercises in Chapter 9. Brain Balance exercises and the nutrition program work synergistically to address all the symptoms in all the systems of the body. If you do not implement dietary changes at the start, you will not get the maximum benefits out of Brain Balance.

GOOD DIET STRATEGIES

Nutrition for adequate development of the body and brain requires a mix of forty-five nutritional elements including vitamins, minerals, amino acids, essential fatty acids, water, and complex carbohydrates. Studies are coming out almost weekly showing that children with neurological disorders, particularly ADHD and autism, have deficiencies in vitamins, minerals, amino acids, and essential fatty acids. Records show that kids eat too many simple carbohydrates in the form of junk and are sorely missing out on complex carbohydrates.

Nutritionists from Purdue University have been working on this problem for more than a decade and have developed some strategies that parents find helpful. As you move on to the next section, the elimination diet, you will want to keep these ideas in mind.

Variety, variety, variety. Variety helps keep meals interesting and, at the same time, helps guarantee that a child will get all of the necessary nutrients.

Go for the grains. Breads, cereal, rice, and pasta are good grain choices that kids can enjoy. A child requires more servings of these foods than an adult. Always go for whole grains, not refined grains. Refined or simple carbohydrates are double trouble in any sensible diet.

Use only good fats. Fat is a requirement for growth. However, the brain needs only small amounts of fat. The brain loves fat, only not the saturated kind that clogs arteries. Opt for healthy monounsaturated fats like olive, avocado, and nut oils. Kids actually enjoy vegetables stir-fried in these fats as they give good flavor.

Think of essential fatty acids as the other vitamins. These nutrients are essential to proper brain health, only the body does not manufacture them. They must be obtained through diet. They are particularly important to children with FDS because studies are revealing a link between shortages of essential fatty acids and the rising incidence of neurological childhood disorders. Rich sources include:

Soy, walnut, and canola oils
Flax seeds
Beans, especially soy, navy, and kidney beans
Walnuts

Tofu

Cold-water fish (salmon, tuna, mackerel, and sardines)

Think more vegetables, less meat. Kids love eating on plates that have separate compartments for meat, vegetables, and dessert. The way to properly fill a plate is to put the vegetables where the meat is supposed to be.

Think outside the meat counter. Protein is important and lean meats should be a part of your child's overall diet. However, keep in mind that protein comes in other forms as well, such as eggs, beans, and nuts.

Be dairy sensible. Kids generally love milk and dairy products, but this is an instance in which a child can get too much of a good thing. Dairy foods are filling, and when children eat too much dairy, they fill up and don't get enough of other important nutrients not found in dairy. Limit dairy to two or three servings a day.

Most children with FDS are sensitive to dairy foods. If you find this to be the case with your child, then you have another issue. Dairy is a chief source of calcium and vitamin D, so without it you will have to depend on supplements. Soy is generally the best substitute if a child is not sensitive to it.

FOOD SENSITIVITY TESTING

Food sensitivities, which are quite common in children with FDS, are insidious because, unlike food allergies, they come on slowly and produce symptoms that you'd never think to blame on food. You have to go looking for them, and I am going to show you how. It's called an elimination diet, something that nutrition and food experts have been using for decades.

You are going to use the same method to help determine if your child is sensitive to a particular food or group of foods. This can't be done overnight or even over a few days. It requires both diligence and patience.

This procedure is going to help you identify:

If your child is reacting to a food and if that reaction is responsible for some of the behaviors you've been seeing.

Which specific symptoms may be related to which specific food.

The severity of the reaction.

How to design the diet.

Parents ask me all the time if food and diet could be related to their child's behavior and learning issues. The simple answer is that there is no proof that food alone is the culprit. For one, it is highly unlikely that food could be the source of the myriad issues that confront children with FDS. I do believe that diet is rarely if ever the primary cause for conditions such as ADHD or autism. However, I do believe that certain foods can trigger certain symptoms and can make the overall problem infinitely worse.

One clue that can be considered a red alert for a possible food sensitivity is erratic behavior. This is the kind of behavior in which a child is good as an angel one day and the exact opposite the next. Or perhaps the child is acting quite normally and then about an hour or so after a meal, all heck breaks loose. These kinds of wild swings are a tip-off that you need to do an elimination diet.

THE ELIMINATION DIET

Ironically, the most common food sensitivities involved in FDS are very nutritious. Dairy and wheat are at the top of the list, so this is where you are going to start. These two foods are also chemically very similar, so it is very likely that if one is a problem, the other will be as well.

There is no reason for alarm if you discover that your child is sensitive to a healthy food. Like all the other symptoms of FDS, the sensitivity will go away once the brain imbalance is corrected. It's also possible that you will discover that your child does not have a food sensitivity.

▶ Step 1. Starting a Diet Diary (7–10 days)

You will need either a notebook or a more formal diet log that can be purchased at any bookstore. You will start by changing nothing in your child's diet. For the next seven to ten days, write down everything your child eats throughout the day. Arrange the diary by meals and snacks and note the approximate time foods are eaten. Write down everything. For prepared foods, check the list of ingredients on the box and write them down, too, if you believe it is necessary.

Also write down all the symptoms your child displays—the time they happen and for how long.

▶ Step 2. Rounding Up the Food Suspects

Review the diary and look for recognizable patterns. Reactions to food sensitivities usually happen anywhere from two hours to three days after a particular food is eaten. Compare the lists of foods and symptoms and see if and how they relate. Use this list of food offenders as your guide. They are repeated here from Chapter 5 for easier reference. Eliminate all foods on the list completely as well as any you suspect from the food diary.

> Anything containing wheat (gluten or gliandin)
> Apples
> All dairy and milk products (casein), including goat milk
> Chocolate
> Tomato
> Corn
> Oranges and all citrus fruits and juices
> Eggs
> Legumes (peas, beans, peanuts, soy)
> Refined sugar
> Baker's and brewer's yeast
> Soy

Make a list of the foods you suspect could be causing symptoms. However, don't be discouraged if you can't see a pattern. This is typical because reactions may take up to three days to emerge, and usually don't produce any obvious physical signs.

▶ Step 3. The Food Elimination Process (4 or more weeks)

This starts the actual eating plan, whereby you will remove all the foods on the above list from your child's diet completely for at least four weeks. However, this is not all that you will be doing. You will now be making a concerted effort to make your child's diet healthier. This part of the eating plan can, of course (in fact, it should for health's sake), include family participation. After you have eliminated all these foods, you will continue with this new program for four weeks.

This isn't going to be all that easy and will require close monitoring. You will need to alert your child's teacher (or whoever can monitor him while in school) and the parents of friends he will be visiting. In addition to the suspects, you must eliminate:

- Junk food—this means all fast food, candy, soda, etc.
- Processed foods—this includes pressed meats and cheeses and most packaged fast-to-the-table foods.
- Food additives—this requires checking labels carefully. The list of food additives is long, and you should get familiar with what they are. They include any ingredients containing the words *agents, enhancer, regulator, gums,* and ingredients ending with *ant.*
- Any other foods that have been detected in testing as a possible insensitivity.

Be aware that your child may go through withdrawal symptoms as a result of eliminating some of these foods. To children with FDS, some of these foods are physically addicting. However, these symptoms should go away within two weeks. They include:

Irritability
Depression
Lethargy
Difficulty sleeping

When the diet is done correctly, you will see a significant improvement in general health and behavior in three to four weeks. If not, it means one of the following:

Your child cheated and ate forbidden food without your knowledge.
The food or foods your child is sensitive to have not been identified yet.
Your child does not have a food sensitivity.
You may not have designed the elimination diet properly. You may need to do it again and include more foods.

▶ Step 4. The Food Challenge

Proceed to this step only if Steps 1 through 3 have resulted in a noticeable improvement. In this step, you will reintroduce the foods that you have isolated for suspected food sensitivities. You will reintroduce them one at a time, but the order in which you do it does not matter. Record your procedure and the results in the food diary. Children with a right brain deficit have behaviors that are usually most noticeable over the weekend, so you may want to start on a Saturday. In children with a left brain deficit, symptoms are usually more noticeable during the week at homework time, so you will want to do this reintroduction during the week. Do as follows:

1. Have the child eat the food at breakfast, lunch, and dinner, increasing the amount with each meal.
2. Record the quantity of the food eaten and the time.
3. Record all the symptoms you observe, the time they occurred, and for how long.
4. At the beginning of each day, make a note in the diary as to the quality of your child's sleep the night before and general behavior the next day (lethargy, moodiness, stuffy nose, etc.).
5. Reintroduce the food for only one day and then remove it again from the diet completely, even if it does not produce any symptoms, until all of the eliminated foods have been tested.
6. Wait three days or until any symptoms are gone for at least twenty-four hours before reintroducing the next food on the list, and test each food, one by one, until all the foods have been evaluated.
7. If your child gets a cold or infection during this step, suspend the process until after recovery. Milk should be considered separate from other dairy products.

If a food challenge results in significant symptoms, do not continue the challenge until all the symptoms are gone for twenty-four hours.

▶ Step 5. Putting It All Together

You should have clearly observed that certain symptoms subsided during the elimination diet and returned when a given food or foods were reintroduced. These suspects should now be considered food sensitivities and should be completely abandoned until after you've achieved success on the Brain Balance Program.

You may notice that you saw a significant withdrawal of bad behavior as a result of the elimination diet but not as dramatic a comeback when the sensitive food was introduced. Consider this good because it is a sign that the Brain Balance exercises that you initiated along with the nutrition portion of the program are starting to take effect.

▶ Sugar and Artificial Sweeteners

If sugar is one of the chief suspects in your child's elimination diet—and it almost always is—you will need to do some detective work to ensure that you are totally eliminating it from the diet.

A no-sugar diet means avoiding all forms of sugar including corn syrup, fructose, dextrose, honey, and maple syrup. Sugar can cause severe behavior problems in children with FDS but taking a child off sugar cold turkey can make the symptoms come back in a few days worse than ever. This, however, is really a sign of withdrawal and the symptoms will again subside in another few days. Even if you find that your child is not sensitive to sugar, you should limit it anyway as you move forward. Sugary foods simply are not good nutrition. Foods that are high in sugar are usually low in important essential nutrients. Also, these foods usually contain artificial coloring and flavoring and trans fats, which you can identify by the words *hydrogenated* or *partially hydrogenated* on labels.

Here are some suggestions to help avoid refined sugar in the diet:

- Substitute fruit juices, drinks, and punches with 100 percent unsweetened orange, grape, grapefruit, or tomato juice.
- Choose frozen and canned unsweetened fruits and pure fruit juices.
- Offer fresh fruits for desserts.
- Use a small amount (a teaspoon) of fruit jams.
- Eliminate sugary cereals at breakfast. A nutritious breakfast should include a high-protein food such as eggs and low-fat milk, as well as fresh fruit and a whole grain cereal or bread.

▶ Artificial Sweeteners

Children with FDS can be sensitive to artificial sweeteners. They include:

Aspartame (Equal, Nutrataste, or NutraSweet)
Saccharin (Sweet 'N Low)
Acesulfame (Sweet One)
Sucralose (Splenda)

Many children diagnosed with ADHD, autism, or dyslexia do not tolerate them well or at all, particularly aspartame. Others can tolerate them in small amount, although saccharin and acesulfame can cause intestinal distress in large doses.

I have found that a child with FDS can generally tolerate several ounces of sugar-free 7-Up, Sprite, or Squirt but only if given on occasion. So save this as a special treat. These citrus-based drinks contain aspartame but no artificial coloring.

You can make a special soft drink soda for your child by mixing club soda with concentrated unsweetened juices to taste. I find that children enjoy it.

All children are different, so you will have to test your child's own tolerance. In general, however, it is best to avoid artificial sweeteners altogether.

▶ Yeast Sensitivities

Candida albicans is a common and usually harmless yeast that lives in the intestinal and urinary tracts. It usually does not produce any difficulty as long as its delicate pH balance (acidity level) is maintained. One thing that can upset the balance is antibiotics.

The problem with antibiotics is that they are so effective, they kill good as well as bad bacteria. In an otherwise healthy child, occasional use of antibiotics is not a problem. However, children with a left brain imbalance tend to get frequent infections, which can expose them to many rounds of antibiotics during their younger years.

Chronic use of antibiotics not only kills the good bacteria necessary for digestion and elimination, it throws off the pH level in the intestinal environment that helps suppress the growth of yeast. As a result, yeast can grow unchecked, causing even more infections and symptoms common in FDS, including fatigue, irritability, hyperactivity, short attention span, spaciness, and depression.

Review the following list of events that are indicative of chronic yeast infections:

Four or more prescriptions for antibiotics within ten to twelve months.
A prolonged course of antibiotics lasting four weeks or longer.
Continuation of symptoms after the infection is cleared.
A craving for sugar.
Persistent digestive problems, including gas, bloating, and constipation or diarrhea.

If you suspect your child has a yeast infection, avoid foods that promote the growth of yeast, such as sugar, honey, corn syrup, maple syrup, and yeast-containing foods, which include breads, dried fruit, and cheese. Talk to your child's pediatrician about a prescription for an antifungal medication, such as Nystatin powder. Do not use Nystatin in tablet form if your child is sensitive to food dyes or as a liquid suspension because it contains sugar. Unfortunately, the only alternative is the powder, which has a slightly unpleasant taste. If your child won't tolerate it, put the powder in clear gels and tablets (you can buy them at any pharmacy) and give the medicine as a pill. Symptoms may also worsen in the first few days but they will subside.

The best natural way to restore the pH balance in the digestive system is with probiotics, namely *Lactobacillus acidophilus*, the culture found in yogurt, and plantarum. You can find these probiotics in tablet form and get them from eating yogurt.

GETTING BACK TO NORMAL

Once the Brain Balance Program takes effect, your child should no longer be food sensitive. This is due to the fact that the immune and digestive systems will correct themselves once the brain is in synchronization. You can start reintroducing the forbidden foods back into his diet.

We do recommend, however, that you reintroduce these foods slowly by following a rotation diet. This way your child can resume eating these foods, but will eat them only occasionally. Kids tend to want to eat the things they like over and over, and parents tend to give them to their kids, just so they eat. This in itself is not good because when the same food is eaten over and over again, it could possibly cause an immune reaction that can lead to creating the sensitivity all over again.

A rotation diet prevents foods from challenging your child's system and becoming addictive. Most of the time, you will substitute sensitive foods with choices from the same food families and then vary the food within the food family over four days.

▶ The Four-Day Rotation Diet

A rotation diet follows a four-day cycle. You'll vary foods within the same food family for four days, then you'll start all over again, repeating the four-day cycle. Use plenty of variety at mealtime to ensure that your child is getting vegetables, fruits, and protein-rich foods daily for optimal nutrition.

▶ Recommendations and Tips

- Read all food ingredient labels and become familiar with the many names a food may be called.
- Many commercially prepared foods and supplements have hidden additives like wheat, yeast, or egg by-products used as fillers.
- Keep a food symptom journal including time, amount, and any changes in attitude, alertness, aches, pains, skin, pulse, hearing, vision, and fatigue.
- Do not feel that you have to follow more than one diet in your household. The rotation diet can benefit everyone by providing variety and decreasing the likelihood of developing food reactions.
- Include at least three different food groups at each meal for variety, satiety, and complete proteins.
- Avoid consuming canned, packaged, and/or fast foods. They contain many hidden, and possibly allergenic, constituents and often lack wholesome ingredients.

- ▪ Unrefined, cold-pressed oils (safflower, olive, canola, sesame) are preferred, as they are less processed and contain fewer chemicals. They also have more flavor. Use organic brands if possible.
- ▪ Get your child to relax and chew, so food is broken down for easier digestion.

▶ Example of a Dairy, Wheat, and Egg-Free Four-Day Rotation Diet

In this example, the child has high reactions to milk, egg, and wheat, so those foods have been excluded completely from the diet. The child has a low reaction to rice and salmon, so those foods are included in the diet, but are eaten only once during a four-day period.

Day 1

BREAKFAST
Buckwheat cereal with soy milk
Grapefruit slices
Banana

LUNCH
Grilled chicken breast with pineapple slices
Green beans
Steamed parsnips

DINNER
Tofu and vegetable (spinach, carrots, celery) stir-fry over quinoa

Day 2

BREAKFAST
Oatmeal with raisins
Chopped hazelnuts
Rice milk
Honeydew melon

LUNCH
Pork chops
Sweet potato
Cucumber salad
Orange juice

DINNER
Scallops and vegetables (bamboo shoots, mushrooms, zucchini)
over wild rice
Watermelon slices
Grape juice

Day 3

BREAKFAST
Amaranth toast, walnuts, butter
Blueberries
Cranberry juice

LUNCH
Salmon
Steamed broccoli
Apple slices and pecans

DINNER
Grilled white fish
Salad of watercress and olives with oil and vinegar
Steamed cabbage

Day 4

BREAKFAST
Spelt toast with apricot preserves
Fruit salad of peaches and plums

LUNCH
Steak with onions and garlic
Asparagus
Baked potato

DINNER
Tomato sauce with beef over spelt pasta
Artichoke
Nectarines

KNOW YOUR FOOD SUBSTITUTES

Dairy foods, wheat, eggs, and molds are difficult to reduce or eliminate from the diet because they are found in many different products. If your child has a reaction to any of these foods, you need to be careful about checking ingredients and also finding substitutes to maintain a balanced, varied diet and a healthy intake of essential nutrients and vitamins.

There are many great sources for food substitutes that can be found in books or on the Internet. If your child has severe food sensitivities, you may want to see a nutritionist or take a class to help you become familiar with common and uncommon ingredients that can aggravate a food sensitivity. Listing them all is beyond the scope of this book.

SUPPLEMENT PROGRAM

Vitamins and minerals are as important to the brain as they are to the body. The minimum daily amount is necessary for healthy brain development. The antioxidants—vitamins A, C, E, and the mineral selenium—are especially important as they help protect the brain from premature aging. It is safe to give your child a multivitamin containing these vitamins in the recommended dosage.

VITAMINS

▶ *Vitamin A*

> *Brain benefits:* Helps protect the membranes of brain cells.
> *Related benefits:* Aids circulation and promotes detoxification in the body.
> *Recommended daily dose:* 10,000 units.
> *Caution:* Vitamin A can be toxic in high doses.

▶ *B Vitamins*

> *Brain benefits:* Essential for the growth and stability of brain neurons. The four B vitamins that are most essential are B_1, B_6, B_{12}, and folic acid.

Vitamin B$_1$ (Thiamine)

Brain benefits: Important for the metabolic processes involving the brain and peripheral nervous system. Also boosts the antioxidant power of vitamins E and B$_6$.

Recommended daily dose: 50 to 100 milligrams.

Vitamin B$_3$ (Niacin)

Brain benefits: Helps in the manufacture of neurotransmitters and converts carbohydrates to glucose. Also has a calming effect on children.

Recommended daily dose: 10 to 50 milligrams as niacinamide.

Vitamin B$_5$ (Pantothenic Acid)

Brain benefits: Critical to the synthesis of the neurotransmitter acetylcholine, which is involved in memory and the autonomic nervous system. Also helps form a protective sheath around the spinal cord.

Recommended daily dose: 50 to 200 milligrams.

Caution: A severe deficiency can produce paralysis.

Vitamin B$_6$

Brain benefits: Helps convert blood sugar into glucose, which is the brain's only fuel. It also improves memory.

Related benefits: Helps boost the immune system.

Recommended daily dose: 50 to 80 milligrams.

Vitamin B$_{12}$

Recommended daily dose: 100 to 1,000 micrograms, depending on age and size of the child.

Caution: A deficiency in B$_{12}$ can result in learning difficulties, poor memory, a decrease in reasoning skills, as well as behavioral symptoms.

Folic acid

Brain benefits: Helps brain circulation. Particularly helpful at breaking down homocysteine, which is toxic to brain cells and nervous tissue. Helps reduce behavior and emotional symptoms.

Recommended daily dose: 500 to 1,000 micrograms.

▶ *Vitamin C*

Brain benefits: Contributes to the manufacture of several neuro-transmitters including acetylcholine, dopamine, and norepi-nephrine. This is why levels are almost fifteen times higher in the brain than they are outside the brain. In one study, vita-min C increased students' scores on IQ tests by an average of 5 points.

Related benefits: If your child has allergies and is prone to colds, vitamin C can help improve resistance. It also improves immune response and protects arterial health. Most children (and adults, too) are chronically low in vitamin C. Many chil-dren with ADD have been found to be deficient in vitamin C.

Recommended dose: 500 milligrams twice a day.

Caution: Possible side effects include gas and diarrhea.

▶ *Vitamin E*

Brain benefits: Helps protect brain cells from oxidative damages and promotes and improves development and function of brain neurons. Studies have shown that, when taken with selenium, vitamin E can improve mood and cognitive function.

Related benefits: Helps arterial health.

Recommended daily dose: 400 International Units.

Caution: Because vitamin E is fat-soluble, it can accumulate to toxic levels.

MINERALS

▶ *Calcium*

Brain benefits: Has a calming effect on behavior.

Related benefits: Critical to bone health.

Recommended daily dose: 500 milligrams as calcium carbonate liquid or chewable tablets.

Caution: If your child dislikes milk or dairy products or is sensi-tive to dairy, it is essential that he take a calcium supplement.

However, too much calcium can decrease the absorption of other minerals.

▶ Magnesium

Brain benefits: Helps the metabolism of neurons. Studies suggest that magnesium has a calming effect on many children with ADHD and autism.

Related benefits: Can help reduce hyperactivity, irritability, sleeping problems, muscle twitching, and bed wetting.

Recommended daily dose: 200 to 600 milligrams as magnesium chloride or magnesium citrate.

Caution: Studies suggest that magnesium deficiency is common in children with ADHD and autism.

▶ Zinc

Brain benefits: Plays an important role in brain metabolism and is part of an antioxidant "chain reaction" that destroys free radicals. In addition, it increases the strength and stability of neurons, and helps to clear the brain of lead, a dangerous toxin to brain cells.

Related benefits: Helps regulate many of the body's metabolic pathways.

Recommended daily dose: 10 milligrams.

Caution: It is estimated that approximately 90 percent of children do not consume the RDA of zinc. If a child has a loss of appetite, slow growth, and white spots on the fingernails, she may have a zinc deficiency. Too much zinc can decrease the absorption of other vital minerals.

▶ Selenium

Brain benefits: Helps prevent oxidation of fats. This is particularly important in the brain, since approximately 60 percent of the brain is composed of certain fats.

Related benefits: Aids the immune system and helps improve circulation.

Recommended daily dose: 100 micrograms.
Caution: Can be toxic in large doses.

▶ *Copper*

Brain benefits: Assists in the functions of neurotransmitters.
Related benefits: Helps biochemical reactions in every cell.
Caution: Excess zinc intake can result in a copper deficiency
when intake of copper is insufficient.
Recommended daily dose: 1 to 2 milligrams.

▶ *Manganese*

Brain benefits: Involved in energy production.
Related benefits: A component of several enzymes involved in
skin, bone, and cartilage formation, and blood glucose
control.
Recommended daily dose: 0.5 to 1 milligram.

▶ *Molybdenum*

Brain benefits: Activates enzymes for building connective tissue
and for removing toxins from the brain and body.
Recommended daily dose: 50 to 100 micrograms.

▶ *Potassium*

Brain benefits: Integral to the proper balance of activity in the brain.
Related benefits: Aids muscle contraction and nerve impulses and
helps keep blood pressure stable.
Caution: Excessive potassium levels in the blood can interfere
with normal heart and nervous system function.

FATTY ACIDS: A BRAIN BALANCE LINK

Not all fat is bad. In fact, fat is essential to brain health. Fat is necessary
for cell membranes, nerve coverings, hormone production, vitamin
absorption, and more.

Most people, including kids, get too much fat in the diet—mostly the wrong kind. Evidence is mounting that there is a link between low levels of essential fatty acids and the incidence of both ADHD and autism.

Good fats in the form of omega-3, 6, and 9 fatty acids are found in foods such as cold-water fish and flaxseed, olive, and nut oils. Make sure your child's diet contains these foods. You can also give your child supplements in the form of fish oil and flaxseed.

▶ *Fish Oil and Flaxseed Oil (Polyunsaturated Omega-3 Fatty Acids)*

This fatty acid begins with *alpha-linolenic acid* (ALA). ALA is an "essential" fatty acid (EFA), meaning that the body cannot make it and it must be gotten from the diet. ALA is converted into *eicosapentaenoic acid* (EPA), which is involved in the regulation of inflammatory processes in the brain. *Docosahexaenoic acid* (DHA) is another omega-3 fatty acid and is integral to brain development in fetuses and infants.

DIGESTIVE ENZYMES

As I explained in Chapter 5, a child with FDS produces fewer secretions in the digestive tract. These secretions include hydrochloric acid and digestive enzymes that chemically help to digest and break down food so nutrients can cross the tight junctions in the stomach and intestines and be absorbed. Children with a leaky gut can benefit from supplementation with digestive enzymes. Once the brain starts to regulate these secretions better, they will no longer be needed. Digestive enzyme supplements can be either an extract of animal pancreas (cow or pig) or can come from certain commercially harvested fungi. The fungal enzyme supplements often have a broad spectrum of activity and are active in a wider range of acid levels. Health food stores and some pharmacies carry a selection of digestive enzyme products. Follow the instructions on the label for children's dosage.

· · ·

BRAIN BALANCE PROFILE: *Alvin*

DEBILITATING DYSFUNCTIONS DISAPPEAR

When we first met Alvin, he was about as far from your average ten-year-old as a kid could be. Diagnosed with both Asperger's at age four and Tourette's at seven, he also had life-threatening asthma, was allergic to milk and wheat, had chronic and debilitating pain at the navel, and had been in speech therapy since the age of three. No surprise, he was also socially withdrawn and not doing particularly well in school.

As if that wasn't enough, doctors had diagnosed him with Gullain-Barré syndrome, a rare autoimmune neurological disorder in which the body attacks the central nervous system. Most recently, doctors had recommended monthly lifelong drug infusions at $5,000 a shot to support his crippled immune system. That was when his parents came to see us.

Despite the fact that Alvin's mom had had him on a special diet since he was six months old, our nutritional analysis showed numerous deficiencies created by a combination of an overreactive immune system and an underfunctioning digestive system. An immediate correction was made in his diet in conjunction with a sensory exercise program designed to address the multiple issues of his right brain imbalance. His parents were both delighted and flabbergasted that within one month of starting Brain Balance, the immune-producing problems that he had endured all his life started to normalize. Before the end of month two, his doctors took him off his expensive "lifelong" immune support. His chronic, debilitating pain also disappeared. Medically, Alvin was like a brand-new boy. His parents and teacher all reported an improvement in his communication and social skills. Testing showed he advanced one grade level (from third to fourth) in his reading skills, though he was still behind his fifth- grade level.

Alvin returned to us a year later for another six months of Brain Balance. Though healthy and happier, he was still struggling academically but making gains interacting with other kids. At the end of six months, Alvin was passing all his subjects for the first time and his school documented him as "a fluent fifth-grade reader with the *emergence of higher order thinking skills." The next month he mastered 100 math facts in his school's 100 Facts in 100 Days Program, and he announced that he wanted to be tested for the gifted program. He now loves science and math, plays the baritone, and recently won the Arrow of Light, the highest Cub Scout achievement award.*

12

HOME BEHAVIOR
MODIFICATION PLAN

Getting Back to Normal

■

Tyler is more focused and more cooperative. When he does act up in school,
the teacher says she corrects him and he stops. Before, he had to be constantly
reminded. I recommend this program due to the simple fact that it works!

—JESSICA H., TYLER'S MOM

■

B EHAVIOR, LIKE EVERYTHING else involved in the brain, has two
sides: good and bad. But every parent knows that! What most parents don't realize, though, is that there is left brain behavior and there is
right brain behavior.

So, if a child has a brain imbalance, as is the case with Functional Disconnection Syndrome, the child's good and bad sides are going to be out
of balance. This means that a child with FDS will not always respond
appropriately to the environmental cues that trigger emotional behavior.
Out-of-sync behavior can be displayed as temper tantrums, meltdowns,
obstinacy, and disobedience. Or it can be seen as being withdrawn, shy,
compulsive, or lazy.

Behavior and emotions are bound together like cement. They are
based in the human primitive instinct for survival—fight or flight. Or as
behaviorists prefer to say, approach and avoidance. Each behavior is
driven by motivation to reach a specified goal, whether it be the desire for
love, warmth, friendship, crayons, or a piece of candy.

• • •

Fight ⟷ Approach
Flight ⟷ Avoidance

TWO SIDES OF EMOTIONS

It's been said that the English language contains more than sixty words to describe emotions but there are only six actual emotions—three fall into the category of approach and three fall under the category of avoidance. They are also broken down into good (positive) emotions and bad (negative) emotions.

Positive (Approach) Behavior	Negative (Avoidance) Behavior
Happy	Sad
Anger	Fear
Surprise	Disgust

Approach, or positive, emotions reside in the left brain, and avoidance, or negative emotions, reside in the right brain. Emotions that are suppressed in one side can be exaggerated in the other. This is why a child with a left brain deficiency can be described as the glum and moody type, and a child with a right brain deficiency can be wild and disruptive. So it only makes sense that for a child to develop the normal, balanced range of appropriate behaviors and emotions, he or she must develop a balanced brain.

Balance in behavior means the ability to respond and act appropriately in any given situation. A child must have the flexibility—the brain signal—to jump back and forth between emotions and behaviors. A child *must be able* to learn what is appropriate behavior and when to behave a certain way. It's important to keep in mind the operative words *must be able* because when a child with a brain imbalance behaves abnormally, it truly does mean that he or she doesn't know any better.

GETTING BEHAVIOR IN BALANCE

Children are born with the same basic drive that all animals are born with—a desire to survive. They develop the more sophisticated goals and motivations that define human behavior and individuality only as their brain, specifically the prefrontal cortex, develops. It is up to the parents to help shape and mold their child's intentions, goals, and dreams, but it takes a balanced brain to pursue and attain them. A brain that is out of rhythm, however, will not develop the emotional structure to carry them out.

It is painful for parents to watch a child withdraw and be alone. It is painful for parents to appear to others as if they can't control their kids. If you are a parent reading this book, you most likely know exactly what I am talking about.

But I have good news for you. The behavior you are dealing with now only seems hopeless and out of control. The Brain Balance Program that you are undertaking is an automatic correction for out-of-control behavior—be it over-the-top actions or just the opposite. Once the brain gets in balance, your child will be in touch with his or her own emotions and have the intelligence to act on them appropriately.

This is not to say that a behavior problem can't be seeded in a psychological cause. It absolutely can. But children with FDS who are the product of a good environment and nurturing, loving parents have a behavior problem that is neurological and can be corrected. It doesn't necessarily require behavioral training; it requires Brain Balance training.

THE RIGHT (AND LEFT) APPROACH

A child with normal left brain behavior is happy, curious, motivated, friendly, loving, and eager to learn. This is the positive side of the brain. A child with a left brain delay can end up painfully shy, insecure, lazy, antisocial, fearful, glum, or even depressed. The child with a left brain imbalance not only has too little approach behavior, but also has too much avoidance behavior. This is what you see with children with dyslexia or a learning disability.

The right brain houses negative emotions, and we have them for a good reason. These are emotions such as fear that will stop a child from crossing a busy intersection against the light. The right brain keeps the left brain from getting out of control—from acting impulsively and inappropriately. It allows a child to act cautiously and sense danger. A child with decreased right brain activity will be hyperactive, oppositional, disruptive, and aggressive. These children can't read people or situations because they have poor nonverbal skills. The typical child with a right brain deficit has too much approach behavior—the classic symptoms of ADHD.

Children with FDS behave the way they do because the area of their brain that controls behavior is underdeveloped. This is the reasoning part of the brain. It's why, as every parent knows, you can't reason with a small child because this part of the brain has yet to develop. It is also why behavior modification programs most often do not work. A child cannot learn a behavior that he or she really doesn't understand.

BEHAVIOR ASSESSMENT CHECKLIST

The following are common behaviors that indicate that your child may have either a left or a right brain deficiency. As before, you will find something familiar in both lists, but if your child has FDS, it will decidedly lean either left or right. Check off those that apply.

▶ *Right Brain Deficiency*

- ☐ Thinks analytically all the time.
- ☐ Has difficulty modeling someone else's behavior, but can do as told.
- ☐ Often misses the gist of a story.
- ☐ Always the last to get a joke.
- ☐ Gets stuck in set behavior; can't let it go.
- ☐ Engages in risky activities.
- ☐ Lacks social tact and/or is antisocial and/or socially isolated.
- ☐ Poor time management; is always late.
- ☐ Disorganized.
- ☐ Problem paying attention.
- ☐ Is hyperactive and/or impulsive.
- ☐ Has obsessive thoughts or behaviors.
- ☐ Argues all the time and is generally uncooperative.
- ☐ Appears bored, aloof, and abrupt.
- ☐ Considered strange by other children.
- ☐ Immature for age.
- ☐ Inability to form friendships.

☐ Inability to share enjoyment, interests, or achievements with other people.

☐ Acts inappropriately giddy or silly.

☐ Has inappropriate social interaction (one-sided social interaction).

☐ Talks incessantly and asks repetitive questions or repeats words.

☐ Had difficulty as a child getting your attention (didn't point to get you to look at or get something).

☐ Didn't look at self in mirror as a toddler.

Total _____

▶ *Left Brain Deficiency*

☐ Procrastinates.

☐ Extremely shy, especially around strangers.

☐ Very good at nonverbal communication.

☐ Is well liked by other children and teachers.

☐ Does not have any behavioral problems in school.

☐ Understands social rules.

☐ Poor self-esteem, especially when it comes to academics.

☐ Hates doing homework.

☐ Very good at social interaction.

☐ Makes good eye contact.

☐ Likes to be around people and enjoys going to parties.

☐ Doesn't like to go to sleepovers.

☐ Not good at following routines.

☐ Can't follow multiple-step directions.

☐ Seems to be very in touch with feelings.

☐ Jumps to conclusions.

☐ Very aware of own clothes and personal appearance.

☐ Seems to be very in touch with their own feelings.

☐ Self-conscious; feels he is being made fun of by others.

☐ Generally very easygoing attitude.

☐ Likes to look at self in mirror.

☐ Difficult to motivate at times.

Total _____

REWARD AND PUNISHMENT

Left brain deficiency: Positive reinforcement
Right brain deficiency: Negative reinforcement

Since all behaviors are built on approach and avoidance, the strategy you must use to contain them is through their motivational equivalent—reward and punishment. If the child makes the wrong choice, then the behavior should be punished in some way, so the child doesn't repeat the behavior.

A child internalizes reward and punishment with different emotions. Reward produces happy, even euphoric emotions, which comes from the brain's release of the chemical dopamine, and the left brain. This feeling can be addictive, so it can drive a child to act a certain way just so he can get the reward.

Punishment comes from the brain and the gut. It causes contractions in the gut muscles that produce a sick-to-the-stomach or pit-in-the-stomach feeling. These are felt in the right brain.

Reward is "felt" in the left hemisphere, and punishment is "felt" in the right hemisphere. This is the key to the strategies you will use to try to maintain discipline and control your child's behavior.

A child with a slower left brain is deficient in reward responsiveness and is overresponsive to punishment. The child with a weak or slower right brain is withdrawal deficient and overly reward activated. So to help motivate a left-brain-deficient child, you must use reward activities. This means positive reinforcement. For the right-brain-deficient child, you use punishment—negative reinforcement. Here's how it works:

▶ *The Left Brain Challenge*

Use the "if you do, you will" approach.

You should give your child with a left brain deficiency a goal that he can achieve and reward him with positive reinforcement when he achieves it. For example, make your child earn privileges like watching television or playing computer games or getting a new pair of sneakers. Punishment and negative reinforcement do not work on a child with a left brain deficit. You must always keep it positive: *If you do* _____, *you'll get* _____. You stimulate with hope.

▶ *The Right Brain Challenge*

To motivate the child with a right brain deficiency, you must use negative reinforcement. This does not mean that you take away something that she has earned—this is not a good tactic. Rather you use punishment as reinforcement. For example, punishment can be no TV or computer time or shopping. It's really all about how you emphasize the situation. Your focus is: *If you don't do* _____, *you will not get* _____. You stimulate with fear. A child with a right brain deficit needs reinforcement that is immediate; if the goal or the punishment is set too far in the future, he will lose interest.

WHAT YOU CAN DO NOW

There are no behavior exercises in the Brain Balance Program. They are not necessary because the behavior will subside once the balance is corrected. I realize, however, that you need to contain your child's behavior as best you can now.

We recognize that there is a lot of emotional turmoil in the life of a child with FDS—and that extends twofold to the parents, who want to establish a pattern of normalcy within the family circle. Because the emotional outbursts and aberrant behaviors associated with FDS are not typical, parents are confused about how to handle them in a way that is corrective and effective.

If possible, enroll in family counseling with a professional skilled in dealing with the behavioral symptoms that your child displays. If it is within your means to do so, it will go a long way in making a behavior modification plan easier to implement. A family counselor can help establish some basic family rules and act as an independent intermediary to foster communication. If this is not possible, there is no reason to despair. The fundamental roots of a behavior modification program can be self-learned. These guidance points are based on the counseling we do with parents in our clinical settings. The only thing you'll be lacking is the professional wisdom and guidance that helps appease a parent when confronted with doubt when something doesn't go as planned or veers dramatically off course.

Most importantly, throw out the guilt and think positively. It is a natural inclination for parents to blame their child's abnormal behavior on themselves. In most cases, this is absolutely wrong; it is not your fault. It is a neurological problem that you have absolutely no control over. You could not have seen this coming. The only control you have is to seek out the proper help, which is what you have done by reading this book.

You now know that your child's problem is fixable. When the brain gets in balance, the exaggerated behavior will disappear. So, hang in there.

"IT'S NOT THEIR FAULT!"

The most common refrain you'll hear from people offering advice and support—professionals and otherwise—is that your child's behavior is not his fault. The majority of professional counselors still stand by the long-ingrained belief that a psychological problem is causing your child to behave the way he does and it can't be helped. So, they tell you that, as the parent disciplinarian, you should not be too harsh on him. This leaves you feeling confused as to what you should do. Now keep in mind that there is much truth to this—there is an unnatural force causing the behavior— *your child's inability to feel his own body*. It's biology, not psychology.

Imagine yourself standing on the roof near the edge of a twelve-story building and not wanting to get too close for fear of falling. Now imagine a friend putting his hands on your back and nudging you to move closer to the edge for a better look. The more you resist, the faster and harder he tries to push. This is similar to what is happening to your child. Because he processes information slower than other children his age, he feels as if the world is pushing him too fast, and he feels that he will fail or fall. Like you on the edge, he becomes oppositional and defiant.

Children who do not feel their own bodies also do not feel their own boundaries, so they *need* external boundaries to feel safe and protected. These external structures must be their parents and teachers. When parents and teachers do not provide enough structure or boundaries, a child will push until he finds boundaries. If he is allowed to behave in an inappropriate way, he will continue to push until someone pushes back. Keep in mind that you are probably dealing with a very intelligent child, so if you give in, your child will know he is being given false boundaries and will continue to push until he feels real boundaries through consistent resistance from both parents. If parents are not united in this effort, the child will learn how to use one parent against the other. This will also confuse the child and increase feelings of anxiety and insecurity.

Children with FDS also require routine and will not transition well if they are being raised in an unstructured environment. Their anxieties and behaviors will only become worse and more exaggerated. This is why it is crucial to carry through on providing structure, no matter now difficult it becomes.

RULES TO RULE BY

In our Brain Balance Center, we coach parents in basic techniques that help provide structure in a positive and loving way. Keep in mind that every parent's experience is different because every child is different. For some parents, these exercises can feel overwhelming. Don't, however, allow yourself to become discouraged because this behavior will not go on forever.

When implementing positive or negative reinforcement at home, keep these precepts in mind:

Be a teacher, not an enforcer. Do not feel or act like someone who is constantly trying to control your child's behavior. Rather, you are teaching your child how to express and monitor her own behaviors by providing her with the proper skills.

Be patient. This approach may be new to both you and your child, so it is likely that parents and child will experience a certain level of frustration, especially at the outset.

Be consistent. The key to learning any new behavior is consistency. So, keep reinforcing positive behaviors and adjusting the negative behaviors by implementing the following strategies. Use them in conjunction with the other Brain Balance activities and you will see positive change results over time, usually within twelve weeks. To some parents, these techniques will seem obvious and simple, but to many, these may be completely new.

These precepts apply to most children with FDS. However, they can be altered to fit the specific needs of your child. Remember, if your child has a left brain deficit, you will implement these ideas by always using positive reinforcement. If your child has a right brain deficiency, you will use negative reinforcement.

CATCH THEM BEING GOOD!

More often than not, children get recognition for negative behaviors rather than positive ones. This is the reason why negative behaviors are so often repeated—they get recognition. And negative recognition, in the mind of a child, is better than no recognition at all.

When a child sees that a certain behavior results in attention, be it positive or negative, the child will almost always repeat that same behavior with the goal of getting attention. However, when children see that a *desired* behavior is being recognized more often than an undesired behavior, then they strive to get recognition by performing the more desirable behavior. In other words, catch them being good instead of always catching them being bad.

As an example, let's take a teacher who walks into a classroom of twenty children; nineteen of them are running around and screaming, but only one child is sitting quietly reading a book. How do you suppose the teacher might get *all* the children to sit quietly at their desks?

Natural instinct might say the teacher will start yelling at the unruly nineteen to quiet down and get back in their seats. Guess what results this reaction gets? It puts the children in control over the teacher! Why? Well, did they have to sit in their seats quietly to get the teacher's attention? No. They simply had to run around screaming.

Now, let's say that when the teacher walks into the boisterous classroom, she loudly and joyfully projects for all to hear, *"I love the way Jim is sitting in his seat and doing his work so quietly!"* What comes next? The nineteen others will scramble to their seats and do what Jim's doing because they want to get the same recognition.

The same concept can work with your child at home. This will take some practice on your part, because it is much easier, and more natural, to react to negative behaviors than it is to take the time to recognize positive ones. However, in the long run you will be very thankful that you took the time to do it.

Now, does this mean that you should ignore the negative behaviors? Absolutely *not*! Which brings us to the next precept.

CONSISTENCY! CONSISTENCY! CONSISTENCY!

If you don't stop _____, *there will be no* _____. *Do you hear me? And I mean it!*

There isn't a parent alive who hasn't used this refrain (Bet you can easily fill in the blanks!) in a raised voice—possibly *hundreds* of times. And was there ever a time when your child didn't stop and you also didn't carry through on the consequences? I'm not a gambling man, but I'd wager the answer is yes. If so, then you'll find this next scenario quite useful.

Let's go back to the classroom filled with nineteen screaming kids and one child sitting quietly and reading. When the teacher walks in and surveys the scene, she notices among the unruliness that one child is aggressively pulling on another child. Should the teacher still address the quiet child first? Absolutely not! The teacher's first obligation is to acknowledge the negative behavior that, if ignored, could put another child in danger. She diffuses the situation and admonishes the aggressive child by saying, "I didn't like the behavior I was seeing so you have lost your privilege to go to recess today." Later, when recess arrives, she's contrite and feels she may have overreacted, so she tells the child, "Go ahead, you can go to recess but I never want to see you put your hands on another child like you did earlier today!"

This is wrong for two reasons. First, the teacher has just taught the child that her words hold absolutely no merit. Second, the child got the message that the only consequence to bad behavior is a little yelling that will be over soon enough. There are no real consequences for the child to internalize.

This very same concept applies to your child at home. If your child thinks even for a second that you will not carry through on what you threaten to do in response to bad behavior, then there is no motivation for your child to display good behavior because you won't carry through on the praise either.

By being consistent and following through from the *first* time you say something, your child over time will see that you really do mean what you say. She will also see that, when it comes to negative behavior, your boundaries are set in stone.

It is so much more satisfying for both of you to hear the praise that comes with good behavior rather than experience the consequences of bad behavior that your child will work at winning the reward. Keep reinforcing the positive behaviors within your child. At the same time, stick to your rules when it comes to bad behavior.

Carrying through on this precept is hard on many parents at first. It can create feelings of guilt, insecurity, and fear that you may not be taking the right approach. But you are. When necessary, reinforce your self-assurance: You *are* doing the right thing by setting and *enforcing* planned boundaries for behavior because you are paving the way for a more productive and successful future for your child, as well as building more credibility for yourself in his eyes.

Being consistent is very effective. Just make sure that the consequence always fits the behavior, which brings us to the next precept.

THINK BEFORE YOU ASSIGN A CONSEQUENCE TO A BEHAVIOR

In the last classroom example, the reasonable consequence for the child's action would be to suspend his recess privilege for the day and make the child apologize to the student he was pushing.

To make this concept work, it is very important that the punishment, so to speak, fits the crime. This means you should think about it in advance—*now*, for instance—rather than the heat of the moment.

This should be easy to do because many of the behaviors you see are repeated, so you are already familiar with them.

Now, sit down and think of the behaviors your child has been displaying recently. Write them down. Think of the appropriate consequences and write them down in a column corresponding to the behaviors. By having these behaviors documented, it prepares you ahead of time as to how you may effectively address them. Here are some examples:

Behavior: Refusing to do chores
Consequence: Left brain deficit (positive)
You'll complete your chores and help your brothers and sisters do theirs as well.

Consequence: Right brain deficit (negative)
There will be no TV today.

Behavior: Fighting with a sibling
Consequence: Left brain deficit (positive)
Play a game together as best friends for the day.
Consequence: Right brain deficit (negative)
You will not have your usual playtime tomorrow.

Behavior: Insults parents
Consequence: Left brain deficit (positive)
You must apologize to parents in front of others.
Consequence: Right brain deficit (negative)
You will clean up after dinner.

NEVER TAKE AWAY A REWARD THAT A CHILD HAS EARNED

This is an important lesson you must learn. Let's take as our example the child who is caught being good in the class of rowdy kids. Over the next several weeks, the teacher catches Jane being good over and over again. The teacher is so pleased, in fact, that she feels Jane has earned a reward of extra time on the computer, which she loves.

Now, let's suppose the extra computer time has come and she sees Jane get into a spat with a classmate she's trying to nudge away from the computer she wants to use. To the teacher's astonishment, Jane even starts to bully the child. Should the teacher rescind the reward? Absolutely not! Jane should not lose the privilege she has already earned, but the teacher can take care of the situation at hand by telling Jane she can take a "rain check"—meaning she can have extra computer time on another day after she has learned to handle her impulses in a more appropriate manner. This way, Jane learns that she must take responsibility for her inappropriate behavior but the reward still stands.

Institute the same idea with your child. The rain check should be a real piece of paper—ours look like a certificate. It is a reminder that your child fully understands that she does not get to take advantage of an earned privilege due to the choices she made on that day. Explain that she will get to use the certificate when she learns to make better choices and take responsibility for her own impulses. This reinforces the learning process for your child that says, *It is worth displaying good behavior because I always get to keep what I have earned.*

When children feel, even for a moment, that what they have earned is at risk of being taken away, it diminishes their motivation to work at being good on a consistent basis. More importantly, children should always be able to feel proud of their rewards so when they do go off course, they understand that negative behavior doesn't get the same results as positive behavior. Which leads us to our next phase in this process.

"HOOK" YOUR CHILD

More often than not, teachers give out tangible rewards that they, or the school, believe thrill children and reinforce positive behaviors. Or so they think. Stickers are a great example. Many teachers will put a sticker on a child's work as a reward for doing the work, no matter how good it is. However, does anyone ever ask the students if stickers mean anything to *them*? In order to motivate children, you must first know what "hooks" them. What truly interests *your* child? The first thing that often comes to a parent's mind is food, usually some kind of sweet treat. But food isn't a good idea, for several reasons. Instead, think of a nonfood interest that is reward-worthy, such as watching a favorite video or playing a certain video game.

Perhaps you're not quite so sure what would be truly motivating to your child. That's okay because it is easy enough to find out. Give yourself a week to observe what attracts your child's attention on her own—not, for example, when she's doing something because another child is doing it. Is it the computer, or a certain computer game? Is it a certain sport, or a certain Disney character? An outdoor activity would be great, because it would get your child outdoors and exercising, exactly what you want her to be doing.

Write down what you observe about your child's personal attractions for a week during the morning, midday, and evening.

At the end of the week, sit down with your child and show her the list you have made. Go over the list with her and explain that until you feel the negative behaviors are under control, the chosen activities will now be considered privileges and not things she can just do at will. Tell her that the privileges are hers to enjoy day to day as long as she continues the good behavior. If bad behavior erupts, the privileges are suspended for the rest of the day. This practice is important because it involves your child in correcting her own behavior. In other words, you are giving your child credit for being smarter than you think! Many parents are surprised at this approach at first, but they also discover how well it works. Taking what hooks your child and turning it into a privilege will save yourself countless hours of wasted energy employing less effective methods to get your child to break habits of bad behavior.

PREVENT THE BEHAVIOR BEFORE IT OCCURS

Yes, preventing bad behavior from occurring in the first place can be a dream come true. You just need the right tactics.

First off, you need to identify the behaviors you want to become a thing of the past. In order to do that, you need to do exactly what you did to discover what hooks your child—document, document, document! Second, one of the most effective ways to prevent negative undesired behavior is simply to inform your child of what is expected of her before you enter a zone that usually triggers a tantrum.

Let's say, for instance, that you are taking your child with you to the library. Before you enter the building, let your child know the kind of behavior you expect. With young children, bend down and get close enough to have eye contact. Then explain in very short, concise sentences that you *expect* (this is an important word to use) that he will use *a quiet voice* in the library because you know—and here comes the positive reinforcement—that he is *smart and knows how* to do it. Also, add that if he feels that he cannot control himself any longer, then you know *he'll let you know* that it is time to leave.

TEACH HOW TO SELF-MONITOR AND VERBALIZE

Almost everyone at some time has been in a situation in which they feel claustrophobic or trapped. Perhaps it was being stuck in an elevator. Or being trapped in an amusement park ride that you couldn't get out of until the "fun" was over. Or being stalled in traffic in a tunnel. Children with

FDS get these feelings all the time because they are consistently in situations in which they are told to behave. In other words, they are told to control impulses that typically want to come out naturally! There is a problem with attempting to do this because these actions are uncontrolled impulses that will happen, well, impulsively, without warning. They can catch both you and your child off guard. This is why it is imperative to teach your child ways in which he can recognize his own behaviors and verbalize his needs accordingly.

You may need to give him some verbal cues at first to help him identify his impulsive behaviors. Most children are actually aware of this; they simply don't have the skills to self-monitor the behavior. For example, in the beginning, you might say, "It's time to leave" when you recognize a behavior coming on.

Self-monitoring is simply the concept of teaching your child how to recognize his undesired behaviors and correct them when they arise. One way in which to do this over time is to progress from using verbal responses, to facial cues, to body language as the means to relay your displeasure with your child's chosen behaviors. You may even need to go from verbal cues to a mixture of verbal, facial, and bodily cues.

This is a form of self-monitoring because it is very difficult for a child to interpret these kinds of cues. Therefore, through repetition and communication, you are teaching your child a very effective way in which to monitor his own behaviors by reading the faces and body language of those around him. These are the ways in which to teach your child how to self-monitor his own behavior over the course of time.

FOSTER INDEPENDENCE THROUGH PROBLEM SOLVING

If you're like most parents, you make the very common mistake of trying to solve every little conflict and behavior issue on behalf of your child. By doing this, you are depriving your child of an opportunity to foster a strong sense of independence.

For example, say your child displays frequent impulsive inappropriate behavior at the dinner table, like jumping up without being asked to be excused and running about the kitchen and dining area. You have several choices in a situation like this. You can:

1. Raise your voice and get yourself and your child into an even more heightened state of excitement.
2. Get up from your seat, walk over to the child, look him straight in the eyes, and give him a small verbal cue how he might solve this issue on his own by saying, *"It's not very polite to jump up from the dinner table like that. Can you think of a better choice to make right now?"*

In response, it is possible for him to:

1. Say, "I could ask to be excused or I should come back to the table and sit down."
2. Respond with a number of inappropriate answers (this includes any type of silly response that has nothing to do with your question) in a voice that exhibits anger or avoidance.
3. Say nothing at all (possibly followed by a physical outburst of some kind).

Here is how you can respond to these actions.

Response: "I could ask to be excused."

Possible solution: Adults who have never dealt with a child with FDS typically say, "But that is not how we do things in our home. The rules are the rules and nobody gets up until they finish their dinner and we spend time together as a family."

Well, let's go back to the example of being trapped in an elevator. What if there was a rule at your office that nobody could take the stairs in the building—that you must take the elevator. One day you get in the elevator and it stops with a lurch and the doors refuse to open. You don't like elevators to begin with, so what happens to your insides? You begin to panic. Your heart starts racing, you begin to move around in the elevator with your eyes frantically searching for the button marked "Door Open." Your breathing becomes very shallow because you are so consumed with trying to find a way out. Your mind is racing with a million different thoughts because your anxiety level has just been raised beyond your threshold. All of a sudden, you find the right button and the doors open. How do you feel now? Relieved, right? What happens to all those symptoms you were having in the elevator before the doors opened? They're gone. You no longer are consumed with finding a way out.

Well, guess what—this is *exactly* what it is like for a child with FDS. Being told that, despite his now polite attempt at telling you he can no longer hold in his impulses, it simply isn't good enough because it's not *your* way. Just like getting to the third floor by taking the elevator. Whether you take the elevator or the steps—you still get there.

What is the goal here with your child? The goal is to teach him to begin monitoring his own behavior by coming up with acceptable solutions to control his impulses. More important, let's look at the anxiety involved in being "stuck" at the dinner table in comparison to being stuck in the elevator. When you force a child with impulsive behavior and hyperactivity to sit still and be "just like other children," you are creating an even *greater* impulse in your child than there was *before* you asked him to sit back down. However, just as in the example with the elevator, if the child learns over time that all he has to do is ask to be excused in a polite manner or simply *verbalize his impulses* by telling you that he needs to get up and walk around a bit before coming back and joining you once again, then all of a sudden, you have just given him his own button to "open the doors" and appropriately "escape" from the situation that caused him anxiety.

Over time, you'll witness that your child's need "to escape" will disappear. Why? *Because you have taken away the element of anxiety.* By doing so, you eventually extinguish the need for your child to act on this impulse because he has the security of knowing that he can verbalize his anxious feelings at any time, as long as it is done in an appropriate manner—the manner that you both learned together.

BRAIN BALANCE PROFILE: *Ellen*

FROM 100% DEFIANT TO 100% CHARMING

Ellen was hardly the picture of health when we first met. She was overweight and had limp hair, a ruddy complexion, and cracks at the corners of her mouth. She also had been diagnosed with ADHD and oppositional defiant disorder (ODD). For a nine-year-old, Ellen was one tough little cookie.

Ellen's mom was the primary breadwinner in the family and worked very hard. Her husband was a stay-at-home dad who took care of Ellen and her siblings. He had ADHD himself and had empathy for Ellen, so he exercised little discipline over the children and provided even less structure in their day-to-day lives. That all changed, however, when Ellen started to fail in school and her teacher called to report Ellen's bad behavior in class and toward her classmates. Mom decided to take matters into her own hands and came to see me.

One look at Ellen told me much of what I needed to know. By her appearance and demeanor, it was obvious that she was sedentary, lacked motivation, and had no self-esteem. I also had a hunch that she had no friends either. (I found out a few months later from Ellen herself that I was right.) She accepted her failure in school as a given—something she expected. "Yeah, so what?" was her response. When we talked, she sounded very anxious and I could tell that she felt insecure.

Ellen also had other issues. She was extremely clumsy, especially with what we call gross motor coordination skills. For example, when she'd put her feet together and close her eyes, she'd fall to the left. Ellen, in fact, had all the classic signs of Functional Disconnection Syndrome. She felt insecure and acted defiant because she didn't feel grounded. This is also why she was so clumsy. Her poor body awareness made her feel unsafe and unsteady. She acted inappropriately in front of others because she couldn't read others' body language and facial expressions. She couldn't relate to her own emotions because she felt disconnected from herself. She was actually very bright but it wasn't readily apparent because she was so camouflaged in the fallout from a severe brain imbalance. Testing confirmed she had a right brain deficiency and we designed a program to correct the problem.

On our first official class day, her ODD was in high gear. She screamed that she hated me and stubbornly refused to do anything I asked. Her behavior wasn't a problem for me—I'm used to it—but I worried about how her parents would respond, especially her dad, who always caved in when she didn't want to do something. You see, one of Ellen's problems was that she had no boundaries, which directly related to her bad behavior. So, I had a talk with her mom. I explained that she needed to be strong with Ellen and eliminate the possibility that she would be allowed to quit. I told her Ellen needed boundaries in order for her to feel safe and secure. She needed structure and stability. Through defiant behavior, Ellen was screaming for boundaries and stability in her life. Children will honor their boundaries, I told her, once they believe that they are real.

As expected, Ellen told her parents that she wanted no part of me and pleaded not to come back to Brain Balance. But Ellen got what she had been needing for a long time—a firm "no."

I can't say that our first few sessions were easy, but Ellen quickly learned that I was in charge. Gradually, she started to cooperate and with cooperation came improvement. As the activities became easier for her to do, she became less resistant and tried harder. Both her mother and I could see physical and emotional improvement. Within weeks, Ellen started to look healthier, was losing weight, and her combative behavior disappeared. But the real report card came when Ellen visited me a few months later. With a big smile on her face, Ellen handed me a sheet of paper—a test she had taken in class that day. She pointed to the grade—100 percent.

Around the same time, Ellen's mom got another call from her teacher, but this time for a different reason. "Her teacher can't get over the big improvement in Ellen. She says she is friendly, participates in class, and is making friends. She said that Ellen's actually a very sweet girl."

13

DEFINING FUNCTIONAL DISCONNECTION SYNDROME

Putting the Left Brain and the Right Brain in Perspective

■

Not only are we NOT seeing a regression
in Matthew, we are seeing continued growth. WOW!
He is more talkative and engaged than ever.

—CYNTHIA, MATTHEW'S MOM

■

JUST AS THERE are two sides to every story, there are two sides to Functional Disconnection Syndrome. Just like the two sides of the story, the two sides of FDS are similar in some aspects and vastly different in others. No matter how you look at it, all children with Functional Disconnection Syndrome generally have two major issues as they are growing up: academic troubles and behavioral problems.

PROFILE OF A CHILD WITH A RIGHT BRAIN DEFICIENCY

A right brain deficiency first shows up as a behavior problem. Mothers often tell me that these kids started giving them a hard time right from the get-go. These are the kids who kicked and moved around in the womb so much that their moms couldn't get any sleep. More often than not, giving birth wasn't easy either. There may have been an unusually long labor or induced labor brought on because the fetus was beyond term.

As infants, these children tried their mothers with breastfeeding trouble and colicky crying. They were fussy babies who were a struggle to get to sleep. But memories of all this trouble are soon countered with parental pride over the fact that these babies seem to be very smart. They delight their parents with fast and early learning. As toddlers, they may pick up a book and try to read it—or actually even read a few words. They hear everything their parents say and have the memory of an elephant.

At this stage of the game, the parents' biggest complaint is that their child seems to be all over the place. These are the kids who run their moms ragged. They can barely sit still for a minute. Nevertheless, they continue to fascinate with their unusual curiosity and fast learning. This is often confusing for a parent because, as smart as these kids are, their first words are often overdue. In fact, they may not speak much at all. However, what they lack in expression, they make up in learning and these children often start school with impressive reading and spelling skills. Unfortunately it isn't too long before that world starts caving in.

Feedback from teachers usually arrives early. Acting out, meltdowns, and obstinate, impulsive, disruptive, and oppositional behavior are among the complaints that parents hear from teachers. Maybe their child will "outgrow" this behavior, the parents hope. At least their child's grades are good. But then that begins to change, too, usually around the fourth grade.

Suddenly, these brilliant children start to struggle in school. They read but it soon becomes apparent that they don't get the gist of what they are reading. They struggle with math. They start losing ground academically, because of all they've missed when they weren't paying attention. Their foundational skills become so weak that their early knowledge base starts to look like Swiss cheese—it's full of holes they can't fill.

Like all kids, they crave friendship but struggle to make friends. No matter how hard they try, they just don't do it right. They invade other kids' territory and say the wrong thing at the wrong time. Other kids just think that they're weird.

This leads to frustration, especially because they know they are more intelligent than most of their peers. As they get more frustrated and fearful, they become more and more oppositional. They usually take it out on Mom first, then go up and down the ladder of authority figures.

These children also have many "sensory issues"—they are either over or undersensitive to the sensory world around them and they tend to be extremely picky eaters.

Mothers often tell me later that they always sensed this child was "kind of different" from other kids. Mothers who have other children say in retrospect that this was the child who seemed "disconnected" early on from parents and siblings. They confide that their child did not display much emotion—even the voice was monotone. Some of these children seem to have problems with just about everything. Unfortunately parents hear scary terms for it: autism, Asperger's, ADHD, pervasive developmental disorder. They become completely overwhelmed.

PROFILE OF A CHILD WITH A LEFT BRAIN DEFICIENCY

A left brain deficiency usually shows up first as an academic problem. So, unlike their right brain counterparts, life for a child with a left brain imbalance starts out quite normally.

Children with a left brain delay do not have the multiple issues we tend to see in right-brain-deficient children. They don't get in trouble in school, pick fights, drive their parents ragged with their hyperactive behavior, or make mealtime unbearable with their fussy eating patterns. At least not early on. In fact, parents generally describe these children as "starting out easy."

Their biggest problem early on is sickness. Chronic ear infections are quite common, and this may have some slight effect on their hearing development, which only aggravates the academic troubles their parents have yet to see.

These kids are fun to watch. They are very coordinated and may even show some early athletic ability. Nevertheless, they can be a bit clumsy when it comes to working with their hands, which is most often noticeable in their dreadful handwriting. This often makes some parents wonder if it is because their child appears to be left-handed or ambidextrous.

These are very spatial kids and they love the outdoors. They love physical activities—they climb, ride a bike, skate, and skateboard. They often show an early ability to handle these skills because they have pretty good balance. However, they tend to shy away from dancing and team sports such as soccer and baseball because they have issues with timing, rhythm, and understanding the rules. These children are often late talkers. However, they tend to compensate for this through exceptional nonverbal communication. Mothers know that these kids can read them and others very well. And they are good little kids who love hanging around Mom and Dad. They might even appear a bit needy.

This loving nature is in sharp contrast to their life once they start school. Children with left brain deficiencies usually struggle in school from day one. They have trouble learning and remembering almost everything. What they learn and retain on one day is often gone the next. They struggle with learning how to read because they don't get it when it comes to sounding out words. They hate to read because it is so frustrating to them. Preschool and elementary school teachers love these children because they are not discipline problems, at least not yet. However, their apparent disinterest in academic pursuits concerns their teachers.

Teachers notice that these children hate sitting still and would much rather be outside playing. These are the kids teachers say are "not working up to their potential." They might even be described as lazy. But this is only because they don't like school. When it comes to things these children do not like to do, they are very hard to motivate. It is not the deliberate or oppositional behavior that you see in their right brain counterparts—at least not yet. They simply have that "I just don't want to" or "I don't feel like it" attitude—and it breeds trouble.

The shift usually begins around the fourth grade when school starts to get tougher. This raises their frustration and tests their good nature. They start to feel that they are "stupid" or "dumb," often because they overhear other kids talking about them this way. They think other kids are making fun of them when they read aloud in class because they do it so badly. They are acutely aware of the way other kids look at them. Some kids have the ability to overcome this with their pleasant personality or athletic skills. (The stereotype of the dumb athlete comes to mind.) More often than not, though, they build up anger and become defiant. This is when you hear from parents that they can't figure out what suddenly happened. Their child, whom everyone loved and got along with, now is a problem child—academically and behaviorally. In come the tutors, the special instructors, perhaps even special education classes. In come the psychologists and behavioral modification plan.

A PARENT'S PERSPECTIVE

At the beginning of the book, I described what it is like being a child with Functional Disconnection Syndrome. The above describes what it is like to be the parent of one. These are generalizations, of course, but they are pretty accurate descriptions.

As you can see, children with a brain imbalance start out differently but they all end up the same. This is what leads to a lot of confusion for parents. However, this is also why one program can work for all of these children so well.

Unfortunately, most parents feel that there is nowhere to turn—that there is no answer to the problem. But you know now that there is. My hope is that every parent of a child with a learning and/or behavior problem will hear about and use the Brain Balance Program.

The sooner you take measures to correct the problem, the easier it will be to correct. The first order of business is to determine what kind of dysfunction your child has—an imbalance caused by a left brain deficiency or a right brain deficiency. This book has given you all the information you need to make this determination. It was presented to you in a logical progression, along with enough of the scientific background to explain how and why these problems occur. You also now have all the tools to fix this problem. And you have the master hemispheric checklist that you can use to periodically check how your child is doing. You will see as time goes on that you will be checking off fewer and fewer characteristics as you move forward.

GOING FORWARD

I have worked with more than 1,000 children during the past fifteen years and have been privileged to see the lives of most of them and their families changed for the better. I never stop getting excited about the results. I got involved with this work not just as a concerned health professional, but mainly as a parent. I have used these activities to make changes in my own children. I relate to parents who are in pain and just want to help their child. It has taken me more than ten years but I finally have come up with a tool that parents who can't afford a formal program can use to help their child. I congratulate you as a concerned parent, and I wish you the best of luck. Let me know how you are doing. You can contact me through my website, www.brainbalancecenters.com. I look forward to hearing from you.

To find a Brain Balance Center nearest you, you can also go to www.brainbalancecenters.com.

To find a professional trained in hemispheric integration therapy or Functional Neurology, go to www.carrickinstitute.org.

To learn more about or to purchase Brain Balance Music, go to www.i-waveonline.com.

This book only represents the beginning of this work. Much more research needs to be done. If you wish to support this research, you can send your donation to the F. R. Carrick Research Institute, where research into these and other neurologic disorders are taking place. For more information, you can call 631-981-1112 or go to the Brain Balance website.

INDEX

Page numbers in **bold** indicate checklists or tables; those in *italic* indicate illustrations.